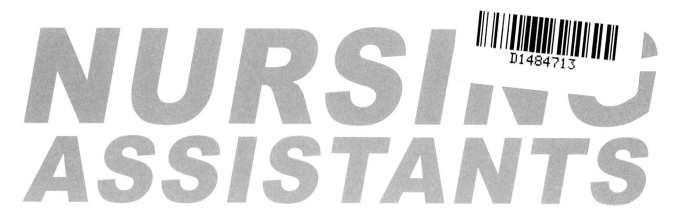

NURSING ASSISTANTS

A Basic Study Guide

12th edition

An OBRA-Specific Study Guide

- to prepare for the certification exam
- to provide in-service training
- to review basics

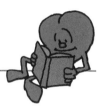

Beverly Robertson, MSC
Kim Price

First Class Books, Inc.
509-276-8000
info@FirstClassBooks.net

NURSING ASSISTANTS

A Basic Study Guide

12th edition

ISBN: 978-1-7923-4899-0

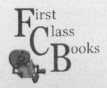

First Class Books

P.O. Box 28493
Spokane, WA 99228-8493

Phone: 509-276-8000
Fax: 509-276-8008
Email: info@firstclassbooks.net

Copyright © Oct. 2020
2018, 2016, 2012, 2009, 2007,
2005, 2004, 2002, 2001, 1998
by First Class Books, Inc.

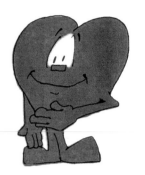

Welcome...

to the honorable career of Nursing Assistant!

Nursing Assistants are the "heart" of long-term care, devoted to improving the quality of life for people in their care. Your skills, along with a caring attitude, will be rewarded with the friendship and trust of the residents, the respect of your employer and co-workers, and personal satisfaction.

This study guide provides core information that is generic for *all healthcare workers*. Although job titles and duties vary (e.g., personal care aides, home health aides, healthcare associates), "Nursing Assistants" is the title identified in the federal regulations that are the basis for this guide. Whatever your title or area of expertise in the healthcare profession, your skills are vital to the quality of life for those in your care.

Nursing Assistants, A Basic Study Guide presents a solid foundation with a positive, friendly approach to learning important skills and procedures. The delightful illustrations add a lighthearted touch to learning the serious business of long-term care.

Acknowledgments

This book is dedicated to those kind, caring, and concerned individuals who devote themselves to quality of life for residents in long-term care facilities. Sincere thanks and appreciation to countless health professionals for their encouragement, support, and technical advice for this study guide.

Contents

Module 1

Being a Nursing Assistant

*Nursing Assistants are
the "heart" of long-term care.*

Objectives:

- Identify duties and responsibilities
- Discuss the importance of the healthcare team
- Describe professionalism
- Discuss professional boundaries
- Explain the importance of confidentiality
- Recognize unacceptable behaviors

Need-to-Know Words:

- certification
- requirements
- practical skills
- clinical skills
- role
- healthcare team
- respect and dignity
- confidentiality
- reliability

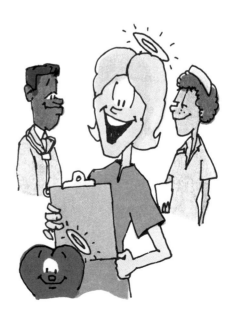

Part 1   Certification Requirements

Certification requires practical and clinical skills.

Federal guidelines establish minimum requirements for Nursing Assistant (NA) training. Additional requirements vary from state to state. Training includes supervised clinical experience in a nursing facility and concurrent (at the same time) classroom theory. Certification requires a passing score on tests for practical and clinical skills. Find out what the licensing requirements are for the state where you work.

Certification requires the Nursing Assistant to understand the following:

- ability to read, write, and understand English at the level necessary to perform the duties of the Nursing Assistant
- NA role and responsibilities
- resident rights

- interpersonal skills
- safety and emergency procedures
- catastrophe management
- body mechanics and lifting techniques
- infection prevention/control
- weights and measures
- care skills and procedures
- vital signs
- nutritional needs
- long-term care
- restorative care
- observation skills
- reporting and charting
- death and dying

Part 2   Role and Responsibilities

Treat each resident with respect and dignity.

The Nursing Assistant provides services for residents under the supervision of a licensed nurse. The job description for the Nursing Assistant varies from facility to facility. Understand the facility's administrative structure and proper reporting procedures.

Depending on where you work, residents may be called patients or clients. This book uses the term "resident" for anyone in a "home away from home." As a Nursing Assistant, you can help make the resident's home a safe, happy, and comfortable place to live.

Nursing Assistants contribute to the health, safety, and security of the residents in three main areas:

- promoting health
- preventing harm
- preventing/controlling infection

Important skills for Nursing Assistants include:

- maintaining a clean and safe environment
- knowing the expectations, limits of the work role, and professional boundaries
- respecting confidentiality
- following directions
- being honest, reliable, and responsible
- upholding resident rights
- showing respect for each resident
- being sensitive to individual beliefs and values
- practicing good body mechanics
- using medical asepsis for infection prevention/control
- being a good listener

- knowing weights and measures
- meeting residents' needs and providing quality care
- recognizing signs of abnormal conditions
- following emergency procedures
- understanding proper nutrition and feeding techniques
- using precautions to prevent infection
- meeting the needs of long-term care
- promoting independence and rehabilitation
- providing comfort and understanding
- being considerate of family and friends
- encouraging recreational and leisure activities
- promoting exercise and mobility
- dealing with death and dying
- practicing personal hygiene
- maintaining your own physical and mental health
- getting along with residents and staff
- developing keen observation skills
- being thorough and accurate
- staying current with skills, including CPR and first aid training

Complete all tasks assigned to you. Tell your supervisor if there is a procedure that you are not trained to do or if you are unsure of how to do it.

Care Team

As a Nursing Assistant, you are an important member of a care team. The care team looks after the total well-being of each resident. The team's goal is to provide the best possible physical care and emotional support.

The NA is likely to spend more time with a resident than any other member of the care team. The team depends on you to provide quality care. Your attitude and skills are very important for each resident's well-being.

The most important member of the team is the person receiving care. Residents are entitled to make decisions about the care services provided for them, and they should be encouraged to be as self-managing as possible. The care team is responsible for providing the best possible care regardless of the person's race, religion, lifestyle, physical or mental condition.

As a team member, you need to understand your facility's administrative structure, policies, procedures, and reporting process. Nursing Assistants work under the supervision, direction, and guidance of professional staff. The care team includes everyone with responsibility for care:

- resident
- doctors
- family members
- nursing staff
- Nursing Assistants
- physical therapists
- respiratory therapists
- occupational therapists
- activities director
- social workers
- clergy
- dieticians
- mental health services

Be a responsible team member. Your cooperation is vital for your team to succeed.

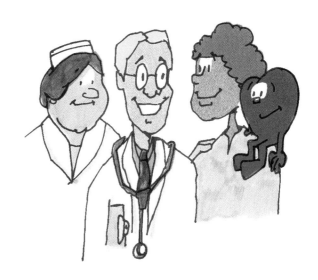

Care Plans

The care team develops a plan of care for each resident. The plan includes any problems, the goal, the approach, and who is responsible for the approach. Carrying out the plan is a team effort.

Before providing care, check the plan carefully and be sure that you understand the directions. Carry out instructions exactly as directed. Total care includes everything that contributes to a resident's well-being:

- proper medical attention
- balanced diet
- exercise
- rest and comfort
- emotional, social, and spiritual support

Part 3	Being Professional

Always treat others the way you would like to be treated.

Always treat the residents the way you would like to be treated if you were the one needing assistance. Your attitude and actions affect how the residents feel about themselves, the facility, and you. Your appropriate behavior is important to the resident's well-being. Always stay within professional boundaries.

Being a Nursing Assistant requires a desire to help people and a caring attitude. Your employer and the people in your care must be able to depend on you.

Providing care for others requires you to take good care of yourself. You need to be well physically and emotionally in order to bring health and happiness into the workplace. Keep yourself neat and clean, and tend to your personal health needs. Try to leave your personal problems at home, and bring a cheerful attitude to the workplace.

Difficulties in your personal life can influence your ability to deliver quality care. Never take out your anger or stress on others (e.g., losing your temper, raising your voice). If you feel out of control, excuse yourself briefly after you ensure the residents' safety and well-being. To relieve your stress, find a quiet place and try deep breathing, talking with a co-worker, or asking your supervisor for help.

Everything you do or say sends a message and affects how people react to you. You send signals by the way you stand or move, your appearance, the way you dress, facial expressions, gestures, and tone of your voice. Always try to send positive messages.

Train yourself to be a good listener and to follow instructions carefully. Ask questions, and remember the answers.

Maintain good working relationships. It is important to get along with your co-workers and to be supportive of each other. Understand the facility's organizational chart, and respect the chain of command. Earn people's trust and respect by being cooperative and professional. Set high standards for yourself, and follow the established requirements and procedures.

Dedication and Loyalty

Being a Nursing Assistant goes far beyond basic duties. You can add to the quality of life for each person in your care. Treat everyone with respect, dignity, and a caring attitude. Promote and support equality for each resident.

Be dedicated to the people in your care, and support the ideals of the facility where you work. Show respect for residents, their families, and staff members (even if you dislike them). Be loyal to your employer, and always follow the policies and procedures of the workplace.

IMPORTANT GUIDELINES
ALWAYS follow these guidelines when providing care.

- Knock before entering a resident's room.
- Speak clearly, slowly, and directly to residents.
- Identify the resident, greet by name, and introduce yourself.
- Explain what you are going to do, and provide privacy.
- Wash your hands before and after every task.
- Follow Universal/Standard precautions throughout all procedures.
- Ensure the resident's comfort and safety.
- Keep the call light/signal within easy reach of the resident.
- Report anything unusual.
- Place used linen, supplies, and equipment in designated areas.

Confidentiality

You have both a legal and moral responsibility to keep all information about residents confidential. Confidentiality applies to all medical information and everything related to personal, social, and financial matters. Never discuss information about residents in public. All records with confidential information should be kept secure when not in use. Whenever you have questions or concerns about confidentiality, talk to your supervisor.

Dependability

Residents and staff must be able to depend on you. Be on time for work, in proper uniform, and well-groomed. If you are unable to work, notify your supervisor at the earliest opportunity (at least two hours before your shift begins).

Perform duties to the best of your ability. If in doubt, request clear instructions. Complete all assignments. Do not skip tasks nor chart records until the task is completed.

Maintain care and security of each resident's personal belongings. Legal actions may result if possessions are lost.

Unacceptable Behaviors

Unacceptable behavior may result in dismissal. Any of these behaviors could cost you your job and your certification:

- using verbal or physical abuse
- stealing or willfully damaging property
- disobeying an order from a supervisor
- neglecting your duties
- altering or falsifying records or reports
- working under the influence of alcohol/drugs
- lying or deceiving

If you have ever been convicted of a crime, contact the state certification office prior to training.

Summary

Certification requires both theory and hands-on skills. Nursing Assistants work under the supervision of licensed nurses. Positive working relationships with residents and co-workers are essential, along with dependability, dedication, and confidentiality. NAs are dedicated to competent care, timely service, and quality of life for each resident in their care.

Review

1. List six or more basic requirements for Nursing Assistant certification.

2. Describe the role of the Nursing Assistant.

3. How does the NA contribute to the residents' health, safety, and security?

4. What is the role of the care team?

5. Identify three or more areas that contribute to total care.

6. Choose one area of professionalism, and describe why you feel it is important.

7. Why is confidentiality important?

8. Identify four or more unacceptable behaviors.

Module 2

Upholding Resident Rights

The NA has a legal responsibility to protect each resident's rights.

Objectives:

- Explain resident rights
- Identify legal issues
- Define quality of life
- Discuss differences in beliefs and customs
- Examine personal beliefs
- Recognize abuse
- Explain how to deal with abuse

Need-to-Know Words:

- rights
- beliefs
- preferences
- legal action
- grievance
- advocate
- reprisal
- individuality
- customs
- abuse
- negligence
- self-esteem
- hygiene
- ombudsman

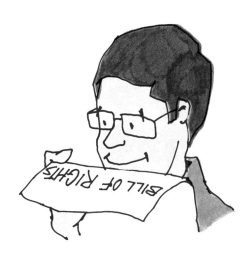

Part 1	**Protecting Resident Rights**

Promote and support individual rights.

Promote and support each resident's rights. Everyone deserves quality care regardless of beliefs, gender, mental or physical ability, background, race, or sexuality. Your personal beliefs and preferences should not affect the quality of service or the way you treat people.

The Resident Bill of Rights is a legal document that protects the residents in healthcare facilities, with an emphasis on dignity, choice, and self-determination. As a Nursing Assistant, you have a legal responsibility to uphold each resident's rights. However, individual rights should not infringe upon the rights of other residents in the facility.

The facility must provide a written description of legal rights. Obtain an official copy of the bill that ensures rights for residents.

Following are examples of resident rights:

- the right to be informed of all rights, before or during admission
- considerate and respectful care
- information about services and charges
- complete information about health status and treatment
- adequate and appropriate healthcare
- free choice and participation in planning care and treatment
- the right to refuse medication and treatment
- notification of significant changes
- advance notice of transfer or discharge and the right to appeal
- the right to voice grievances and file complaints without interference or reprisal
- prompt efforts to resolve grievances
- established visiting hours

- freedom from abuse, neglect, or mistreatment
- confidentiality of personal and clinical information
- management and security of personal funds
- freedom from any physical or chemical restraint, unless agreed to by the resident, ordered by the doctor, and necessary to protect the resident
- the right not to perform services for the facility unless the services are part of the resident's therapeutic care plan and the resident consents

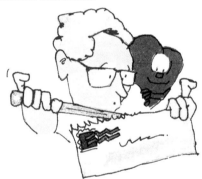

- the right to send and receive mail promptly that is unopened
- access to private use of a telephone
- participation in resident and family groups
- interaction with people in the community
- participation in social, religious, and community activities
- the right to keep and use personal belongings
- the right to private visits with spouse or to share a room with resident spouse
- equal access to quality care regardless of source of payment

In addition to meeting their basic needs, residents have rights to quality of life, focusing on resident-centered care that enhances each person's dignity and self-esteem (personal pride). Care is based on each resident's strengths, needs, and preferences.

Welcome new residents and help them adjust as soon as they are admitted to the facility. Familiarize residents and their families with the facility and services. Show them where things are and how to use them (e.g., telephones, toilets, nursing stations, call lights/signals).

The facility has requirements to ensure resident rights. For example, an ombudsman is an impartial person who investigates complaints and acts as an advocate for residents and/or families to resolve conflicts.

Following are other examples of requirements:

- adequate staff
- food of the quality and quantity needed
- a call system that is easily accessible at all times
- good personal hygiene (including measures to prevent pressure ulcers and prevent/reduce incontinence)
- ongoing activities that are staffed and equipped to meet interests and needs
- homelike environment that is safe, clean, and comfortable
- adequate lighting, safe and comfortable temperature, good ventilation, and appropriate sound levels

Part 2 — Respecting Individual Beliefs

Recognize and support individual beliefs and preferences.

Actively encourage people in your care to express their beliefs, wishes, and views, as long as they do not interfere with the rights of others. Respond in a manner that is supportive.

Beliefs and Preferences

Acknowledge individual beliefs about self, religion, politics, culture, ethics, and sexuality. Beliefs and preferences affect many activities of everyday life:

- foods a person eats
- how a person worships
- values and ethics
- interactions with others
- clothing preferences
- feelings about death and dying

It is important to recognize and accept others' beliefs and lifestyles, even if they clash with your own. Every person has the right to quality of life, regardless of age, gender, physical or mental ability, race, culture, religion, beliefs, or lifestyle.

Following are ways to support individual beliefs.

- Be sensitive to each person's needs.
- Support the right to practice individual beliefs, and respect each person's customs and possessions.
- Make sure your speech and actions do not offend anyone.
- Address individuals in their preferred manner (title, name, nickname).
- Consider beliefs and lifestyles when taking part in care planning.

- Show interest in each person's beliefs.
- Be willing to listen when a resident wants to talk.
- Never question or make fun of another's beliefs.
- Never try to force your beliefs on anyone.

Carefully examine any feelings of hostility. Your personal beliefs affect your behavior in a variety of direct and indirect ways. Never allow your beliefs to interfere with the quality of service for anyone in your care.

Learn all you can about religions, customs, and beliefs, including practices of ethnic minorities in your local area. Ask people to tell you about their beliefs and traditions, or go to the local library for information.

Religious Customs

Be familiar with religious customs. The more you know, the less likely you are to accidently offend someone. People may have religious items in their rooms (such as rosaries or prayer books). If you must move these items, handle them with respect.

Never place items on top of Bibles or other religious books or religious articles. Take special care if religious medallions are pinned to pillows or clothing.

Holidays and Rituals: Be aware of days that are celebrated with special rituals. People may need extra help dressing for holidays, or they may need privacy for certain rituals (such as confession or prayer).

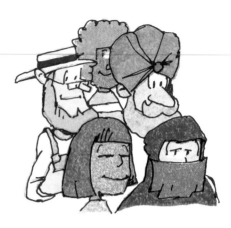

Clothing: Some religions have certain articles of clothing that should be treated with respect.

Foods: Some religions forbid certain foods. Know what is not allowed and offer other choices. Be aware of special times that people may fast (go without food) or eat only certain foods.

Medical Treatments: Be aware of any medical treatments that are not allowed because of religious beliefs.

Clergy: If a person wants to see a clergy member, make sure your supervisor is informed. Provide privacy whenever a clergy member visits.

Part 3   Protecting Individuals from Abuse

Report all complaints and any suspected abuse.

Anyone who cares for the elderly must learn to recognize the various forms and signs of elder abuse. Careful observation is extremely important. Failure to report any suspected abuse or neglect is grounds for legal action. Reporting is mandatory to protect the rights of the resident. Be knowledgeable of your state's requirements regarding mandatory reporting of abuse or neglect.

Abuse is any physical or mental mistreatment of a resident. It includes neglecting basic needs, failure to provide needed care, services, or supervision—whether deliberate or due to carelessness. If you have reasonable cause to believe there is an issue, trust your feelings and follow the reporting procedures for the facility where you work. By intervening promptly, you can prevent suffering and further harm.

Following are legal definitions of abusive behavior:

abuse: mental, physical, sexual, medical, or financial exploitation

assault: an unlawful personal attack

battery: an attack where an actual blow is delivered

negligence: failure to give assigned care, or giving improper care that causes harm

false documentation: entries in a person's record that are not true or have been altered

defamation: falsehoods that result in damage to a person's reputation or character

(libel: a written statement)

(slander: a spoken statement)

If you observe abuse or neglect by anyone, you must report it. Otherwise you will be held responsible and may be subject to dismissal. Be alert to possible abuse, and report any unexplained injuries or sudden behavioral changes. Some residents are unable to speak for themselves. They may need you to be an advocate (spokesperson or representative) for them.

Indicators of possible abuse include the following:

- burns, bruises, lacerations
- torn, stained, or bloody underclothing
- difficulty walking or sitting
- agitation, anxiety, fear, anger
- withdrawn, confused, depressed

Indicators of possible neglect include the following:

- contractures, pressure ulcers
- dehydration, malnutrition, impaction
- poor hygiene, body odors
- change in appetite, weight

If a resident has a complaint, or you suspect something is wrong, tell your supervisor immediately. Make a detailed written report.

Following are examples of abuse and neglect:

- forcing, threatening, calling names
- making fun of a resident
- using restraints without doctor's orders
- inappropriate touching in a sexual manner
- pushing, pinching, unnecessary roughness
- forcing utensils into the resident's mouth
- failing to provide appropriate care
- not following the plan of care
- failing to feed a resident or provide fluids

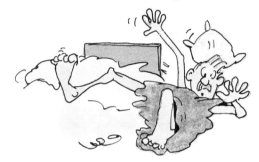

- not raising bed rails when ordered, leading to someone falling from bed
- serving the wrong meal
- failure to reposition a resident, leading to complications
- not responding to a call light/signal

If you have any concerns about dealing with abuse, seek advice from an appropriate person.

Summary

Nursing Assistants have a legal obligation to uphold residents' rights and to protect them from physical and mental harm. Each resident is entitled to quality of life that enhances the person's dignity and self-esteem. Quality care respects individual beliefs and focuses on individuality, strengths, needs, and preferences.

Review

1. Identify six or more resident rights.

_____

_____

_____

_____

2. Why is it important to understand an individual's beliefs and preferences?

_____

_____

_____

_____

3. Identify five or more ways you can support an individual's beliefs.

_____

_____

_____

_____

4. What should you do if a resident complains about the facility?

_____

_____

_____

5. Give five or more examples of abuse.

_____

_____

_____

_____

6. Explain legal responsibilities related to resident care.

_____

_____

_____

_____

7. What is false documentation?

_____

_____

_____

_____

8. Describe three or more examples of neglect.

_____

_____

_____

Developing Interpersonal Skills

Help the residents feel good about themselves and reach for their dreams.

Objectives:

- Identify basic needs
- Demonstrate ways to develop positive relationships
- Recognize the concerns of residents
- Use effective communication skills
- Discuss emotional barriers
- Recognize defensive behavior
- Communicate with residents who are physically impaired

Need-to-Know Words:

- interpersonal
- basic needs
- verbal
- nonverbal
- feedback
- paraphrase
- compassion
- barriers
- significant others
- sexuality
- empathy
- defensive behavior
- visually impaired
- hearing impaired
- cognitively impaired
- aphasia

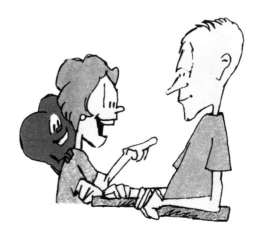

Part 1   Understanding Basic Needs

Unmet needs affect people physically and emotionally.

Everyone has basic needs. When the basic needs are not met, people are affected physically, emotionally, mentally, and socially. Common reactions to unmet needs are depression, anxiety, fear, anger, hostility, withdrawal, and physical ailments.

A psychologist named Abraham Maslow identified steps for meeting needs in his Hierarchy of Human Needs. The illustration on this page identifies Maslow's five "steps" and examples for meeting each need.

A person's needs must be satisfied at one level before moving upward in a step-by-step progression from basic physical needs toward self-actualization. The NA plays an important role in meeting the resident's needs.

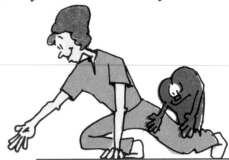

Self-actualization
(reaching for dreams)
- Be enthusiastic and supportive.
- Encourage projects and plans.
- Acknowledge accomplishments.
- Be positive about the future.
- Promote optimism.

Self-esteem
(pride)
- Encourage independence.
- Be supportive.
- Praise when appropriate.
- Welcome ideas and suggestions.
- Ask for opinions.
- Help residents look their best.
- Respect beliefs and belongings.
- Treat residents with dignity.
- Make residents feel worthwhile and important.

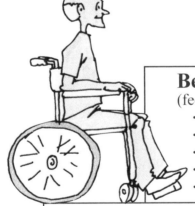

Belonging
(feeling accepted)
- Show that you care.
- Promote interaction with others.
- Listen attentively.
- Be patient and kind.
- Make residents feel "at home."
- Show respect for family and friends.
- Support beliefs and values.
- Respect individuality.
- Allow choices whenever possible.
- Respect privacy and confidentiality.
- Establish trust.

Safety and Security
(safe from harm)
- Provide safe surroundings.
- Be alert to potential hazards.
- Know emergency procedures.
- Keep call light/signal within easy reach.
- Respond to call light/signal quickly.
- Maintain confidentiality.
- Observe and chart accurate information.
- Report anything abnormal.

Physical
(survival requirements)
- Provide quality care and comfort.
- Deliver correct food tray to each resident.
- Assist with feeding as necessary.
- Supply fresh water, and encourage fluids.
- Use precautions to prevent infection.
- Assist as needed with elimination.
- Position for easy breathing, and reposition often.
- Report physical changes.
- Tend to physical needs.
- Reposition frequently.

Part 2 — Building Relationships

The way you treat residents affects their behavior and how they react to you.

Quality care goes beyond meeting a resident's physical needs. Everyone needs a sense of belonging and self-worth. Follow these guidelines to establish good working relationships.

Get off to a good start. You can start building a good relationship when a new resident is admitted to the facility. Keep in mind that this may be a very stressful time for the resident and the family. Be as supportive and helpful as possible. Introduce yourself, and explain that you are there to help. Familiarize newcomers with the facility, and make them feel at home. Introduce roommates and other residents as appropriate. Follow the facility's admissions procedures.

Be kind, caring, and courteous. Whenever a resident needs your help, be patient and supportive. Be pleasant to the resident's family and friends, and make them feel welcome. Invite them to help with basic care of the resident as permitted. Many people do not wish to be called by their first names. Ask how each person wants to be addressed, and greet them by name. Always be courteous and show respect.

Respect individual values, beliefs, and preferences. As a Nursing Assistant, you will care for people whose culture, traditions, beliefs, and values are different from yours. Be sensitive to the differences without being judgmental. Show respect for each resident's lifestyle and his or her religious, cultural, and social practices. Support each resident's rights and consider each person's needs and wishes.

Provide a safe and comfortable environment. Be alert to safety hazards, and protect the residents from harm. Offer warmth and caring to help each resident feel protected and safe. Provide adequate ventilation, quiet, light, and appropriate room temperature.

Always knock before entering a resident's room. Remember the room is the resident's living quarters.

Provide the privacy and courtesy you would show to people in their own homes.

Introduce yourself. Some residents have difficulty remembering names. Say your name whenever you enter the room to avoid confusion or embarrassment for the resident.

Take time to listen. Get to know each person in your care. Value everyone's opinion. Find out about each person's interests and hobbies, and promote activities based on the person's specific interests and abilities. Actively listen and observe body language to gain valuable insights into each resident's needs and expectations.

Encourage friendships. Promote social activities and interaction with other residents. Assist residents if they need help getting to and from activities.

Offer choices. Choices encourage independence. If your schedule permits you to give a resident a bath now or in 30 minutes, let the resident choose. Be specific in your options, and stick to your promises. If a request cannot be granted, explain why.

Be supportive when residents are transferred or discharged. Change can be very stressful. Prepare for the move according to your supervisor's instructions and facility procedures. Make transferring and discharging as smooth as possible for residents and their families. Let residents know you care about them and will miss them.

Significant Others

Significant others are relatives, friends, and anyone who is important to another person. Know who is significant to the people in your care.

Assist residents with sending and receiving letters and messages. Help arrange visits if possible, and provide a setting that is appropriate for visiting. Loved ones offer valuable emotional support for residents. Encourage visitors to participate in care whenever appropriate (with the resident's approval). Provide any training that is necessary.

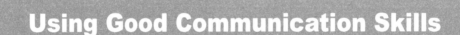

Make visitors feel welcome. Listen attentively, but do not get involved in family matters.

Always remember that information about the resident is confidential. Refer visitors to your supervisor if you are unsure about answering their questions. If you must give care when visitors are present, politely ask visitors to leave the room, and let them know when they can return. Maintain the resident's privacy and dignity at all times.

Sometimes significant others are angry or upset about the illness of their loved one. Even though it may be difficult for you, be patient, understanding, and supportive of significant others.

Sexuality

Regardless of age, humans are sexual beings with sexual thoughts and desires. The NA must deal with sexuality in a mature and professional manner. Respect the need for privacy. Do not interfere with consenting partners as long as no one is in danger of physical harm. If problems arise, ask your supervisor how to handle the situation.

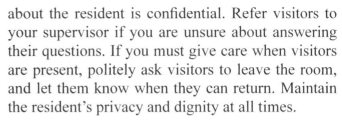

Part 3   Using Good Communication Skills

Everything you do or say communicates a message.

Good communication skills are essential. Speaking, listening, feedback, and actions are important for everything a Nursing Assistant does:

- providing proper care, following directions
- showing concern, building trust
- getting along with residents, families, visitors, and co-workers
- reducing conflict, solving problems
- reporting observations, giving clear messages
- listening, not interrupting or judging
- explaining procedures, resolving concerns
- building relationships

Communication simply means sending and receiving messages. However, effective communication involves more than words. Both verbal and nonverbal messages carry meaning.

Verbal. *Words.* Use simple and clear words.

Nonverbal. *Body language.* Everything you do sends a message:

- facial expressions
- gestures
- tone of voice
- posture
- eye contact
- silence
- touch

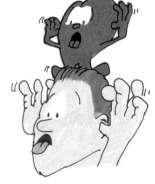

Verbal and nonverbal language must agree in order to send clear messages. The problem is that most people are not aware of their nonverbal behavior. Unless verbal and nonverbal language agree, the listener gets a mixed message. For example, if the NA expresses care and concern, but stands with folded arms and a look of disgust, the resident gets conflicting messages. Unfortunately, when messages are mixed, the nonverbal impressions speak louder than the words.

Communicate as clearly as possible to avoid any confusion. Medical abbreviations are important for NAs to know in order to understand instructions. But do not use abbreviations when you are talking with the residents or their families. Use words that are easily understood.

Listening

Active listening takes effort, self-control, and practice. Pay attention to what the other person is saying, and fight the tendency to think about your reply while the other person is talking. Avoid interrupting or finishing someone else's sentences. Teach yourself to be patient and wait for your turn to talk.

Residents need to feel listened to, heard, and understood. Listen for facts and listen for feelings. Ask questions when you do not understand. Being a good listener helps the NA learn what the resident likes and doesn't like, as well as problems, concerns, interests, and needs.

Feedback

Words have different meanings to different people, which can lead to misunderstandings. Feedback is a process to avoid confusion and to clear up any misunderstanding.

To be sure that you understand what others say to you, paraphrase (repeat what you heard using your own words). Ask if the statement is correct. Check whether others understand what you are saying by asking questions and encouraging feedback.

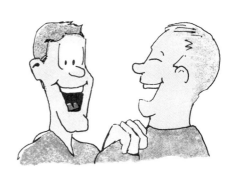

Guidelines for Effective Communication

Open your heart to the residents, and try to understand their problems, pain, and frustrations. Try to imagine what it is like to be in their situation. Take time to smile and say "hello." Convey warmth, understanding, and interest. Small acts of kindness can brighten someone's day.

Communicate with people at their level of understanding. Use an appropriate manner, level, and pace according to individual abilities.

- Take time to listen.
- Be patient, and show respect.
- Think before you speak.
- Be aware of your body language.
- Speak clearly, and use a friendly tone.
- Use simple words and short sentences.
- Ask open questions (e.g., "how?" or "why?").
- Paraphrase (summarize in your own words).
- Ask for clarification.
- Be alert to key words about feelings (e.g., "guilt" or "hurt"), and ask for more information.
- Avoid criticizing or judging.
- Do not interrupt.

Good communication skills build positive relationships. Keys to maintaining good relationships include kindness, caring, and understanding.

| Part 4 | # Dealing with Difficult Behavior |

Behavior may disguise a resident's need for comfort and understanding.

Recognizing the link between actions and needs helps build good relationships. Keep in mind that residents in long-term care are adjusting to changes in their lifestyles that affect them physically, emotionally, and socially.

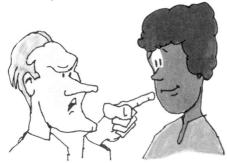

Difficult behavior may signal a need for comfort and understanding. Or it may be an attempt to be in control when a person feels powerless. For example, rather than being annoyed when a resident continually uses the call light, stop by often to offer reassurance.

Basic psychological needs are the root of most conflict. Following are four basic needs identified by Dr. William Glasser for motivating behavior.

Belonging:	loving, sharing, cooperating
Power:	achieving, accomplishing, being recognized and respected
Freedom:	making choices
Fun:	laughing and enjoying

Difficult behavior is a symptom of a problem (e.g., anger, fear, boredom, loneliness). Look beyond the behavior for possible unmet needs. Try to recall any incidents that might have triggered an outburst in order to avoid future problems.

In difficult situations, stay calm and reassuring. Pay particular attention to your voice (tone and volume), your posture, facial expression, and other nonverbal signals. Be willing to listen to concerns, and assure residents that you care about them.

Coping with changes can be difficult for anyone. The elderly face significant changes that can bring a sense of loss, loneliness, frustration, fear, depression, lack of self-confidence, and many other unpleasant feelings. If a resident seems upset, ask how you can help, and take time to listen.

Consider some of the concerns that affect the elderly, and show compassion (sympathy for another's suffering):

- change in lifestyle, loss of independence
- health problems, pain, unable to sleep
- unmet physical and social needs
- longing for the "good old days"
- loss of loved ones
- confusion
- loneliness
- lack of control
- financial concerns
- family problems
- facing mortality (death)

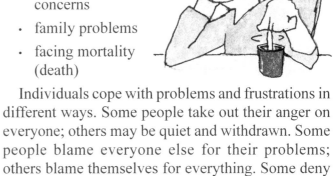

Individuals cope with problems and frustrations in different ways. Some people take out their anger on everyone; others may be quiet and withdrawn. Some people blame everyone else for their problems; others blame themselves for everything. Some deny there is a problem; others try to find a reason or excuse for everything.

Sometimes residents are uncooperative, demanding, threatening, rude, stubborn, or unpleasant. Do not argue or feel hurt. Be calm and supportive. Try to look beyond the behavior to the underlying need for comfort and understanding. Identify and encourage coping skills that help the resident (and you) deal with difficult situations.

Resolving Conflict

Being a Nursing Assistant requires a sincere desire to help others and a genuine interest in the sick and aged. You must be able to treat all people with dignity, including people with physical, mental, or emotional problems. Being a Nursing Assistant can be stressful and demanding, both physically and mentally. To stay motivated and to provide quality care, keep a positive attitude and take good care of yourself. Leave personal problems at home, and leave work-related issues at work.

Your attitude affects the behavior and well-being of the residents as well as your co-workers. It is to everyone's benefit to resolve any conflict that arises in the workplace. If conflict is not resolved, it breaks down relationships, increases negativity, and decreases productivity.

The key to resolution is to identify the conflict before it spins out of control. Then attack the problem and find compromises, as you work toward a win-win solution.

Listen, without interrupting, and try to understand the other person's point of view before defending your position. Pay attention to your nonverbal communication (e.g., look the person in the eyes without glaring, avoid folding your arms). Never jump to conclusions or assume you know what the other person is feeling. Use feedback to gain clear understanding of each other. Explore options together, discuss necessary changes, and identify possible solutions. Never express anger toward the residents or your co-workers. If necessary, find a quiet place until you are in control of your feelings.

Do not let your ego get in the way of resolution. Stay positive, and focus on the present and future, including your needs. Do not dig up the past. Attack the problem, not each other, as you discuss areas of common interest and agreement. If the conflict cannot be resolved, ask your supervisor for advice.

Part 5 — Dealing with Emotional Barriers

Set your feelings aside, and always provide the best possible care.

Good interaction with the residents is vital. Emotional barriers can block communication and prevent positive interaction. As a Nursing Assistant, it is important not to let your feelings interfere with providing the best possible care for each resident.

Everyone has the same basic needs, but each person is different than anyone else. Differences in the way people look, think, or behave sometimes cause misunderstandings, fear, or frustration. You may have negative feelings about certain beliefs, religions, races, cultures, backgrounds, or experiences. Regardless of your personal feelings, each resident has the right to quality care.

Listen to residents with an open mind. Respond to problems or complaints in a caring and courteous manner. Supportive feedback strengthens self-esteem and builds good relationships. Following are examples of caring responses to problems and concerns.

"Tell me more about the problem."

"How can I help?"

"You seem upset, and I want to help you."

Avoid being defensive. People tend to lash out whenever anything threatens their self-esteem. Defensive behavior can destroy relationships and affect work performance. Respond to hurtful comments in a calm and controlled manner. Try to resolve issues without feeling angry or hurt. If you make a mistake, admit it, learn from it, and move on.

If your supervisor offers suggestions, accept the comments without feeling defensive or making excuses. Constructive feedback is an opportunity to improve your work performance.

Make residents feel good about themselves, and avoid situations that make them feel defensive. Create an atmosphere in which residents feel accepted and confident to talk freely about their thoughts and feelings.

Consider your attitude toward illness and health care. As a Nursing Assistant, you will interact regularly with people who depend on you for physical and emotional care. If you enjoy helping people, being a Nursing Assistant is very satisfying. If not, you should consider another career for your own sake as well as the residents' well-being.

Avoid the following behaviors that are emotional barriers to communication:

- acting impatient, irritated, or annoyed
- ignoring, acting bored
- threatening, shouting, or using harsh language
- judging or giving advice
- arguing
- interrupting
- changing the subject
- belittling
- being defensive

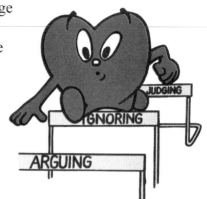

Part 6   Overcoming Physical Barriers

Consider each person's needs and level of understanding.

Nursing Assistants provide care for people with physical disabilities. Problems with seeing, hearing, or mental impairment can be barriers to communication. Speak face-to-face whenever possible. The following guidelines will help you interact with residents who have physical barriers.

Visually Impaired

Follow these guidelines to communicate with people who have difficulty seeing.

- Get the person's attention before talking.
- Identify yourself when entering the room.
- Explain what you are doing.
- Ask for feedback to check for understanding.
- If the resident has eyeglasses, encourage the person to wear them. Help clean the glasses if needed.

Hearing Impaired

Follow these guidelines to communicate with people who have difficulty hearing.

- Gain the person's attention before talking.
- Eliminate unnecessary noises.
- Get close to the person and speak loudly enough to be heard without shouting.
- Maintain eye contact; avoid turning or looking away while you are talking.
- Make sure you face the resident who reads lips.
- Speak to the side where hearing is best.
- Use gestures.
- Ask for feedback to determine understanding.
- If necessary, use paper and pencil to write messages.
- If the resident has a hearing aid, encourage him or her to wear it. Be sure it is clean and working.

Cognitively Impaired

People who are cognitively impaired have difficulty processing information. Communication must be simple, using basic words and short sentences.

Ask for ongoing feedback to be sure the person understands what you said. You might ask the person, "Tell me what I just said," or, "Do you understand me?" Follow these guidelines to communicate with people who are cognitively impaired.

- Use words that are simple and specific.

- Speak slowly and clearly.

- Break information into small parts.

- Try to relate what you say with information the person already knows and understands.

- Treat the person with respect, and repeat the information if necessary (or present the same information in a different way).

- Check often to be sure the person understands what was said.

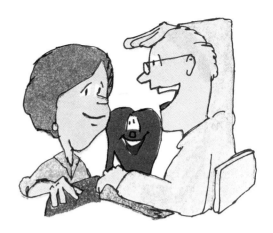

- Use nonverbal aids such as gestures, pictures, paper and pencil, drawings, demonstrations, message board.

- Be supportive and positive, avoiding criticisms/corrections.

- Talk normally. Do not "talk down" to the person or speak too loudly.

- Ask the person to repeat if necessary, rather than pretending you understand.

Your actions communicate a clear message to residents—whether or not they can see, hear, or process information. Be sure your actions send the message that you care about the residents. Always treat them with kindness, dignity, and respect.

Aphasia

Aphasia is partial to total loss of the ability to communicate (verbally and/or written words). Injury or disease can damage the area of the brain that affects language, making communication difficult and frustrating. Follow these guidelines to communicate with aphasic people.

- Address the person by name.

- Eliminate unnecessary background noises (to help the resident concentrate on what is being said).

- Speak slowly and use simple words.

- Ask questions that can be answered with yes or no.

- Be patient, allowing time to process the information and for response.

- Make the message clear, emphasizing key words, limiting details.

Summary

Ensure each resident's basic needs are met. Provide a safe, caring, and comfortable environment. Welcome visitors and treat them with respect. Learn appropriate communication skills to build positive relationships and to overcome physical and emotional barriers. Keep a positive attitude, and ask for help in difficult situations or when you feel overwhelmed.

Review

1. Why is it important for the NA to understand basic needs?

_____

_____

_____

_____

2. Identify three or more basic needs.

_____

_____

_____

_____

3. Identify five or more ways you can build positive relationships with residents.

_____

_____

_____

_____

4. Why should you knock before entering a resident's room?

_____

_____

_____

_____

5. Explain some underlying causes of difficult behavior.

_____

_____

_____

_____

6. Why are good communication skills important?

_____

_____

_____

_____

7. List six or more guidelines for good communication.

_____

_____

_____

_____

8. Describe nonverbal communication.

_____

_____

_____

_____

Module 4

Using Good Body Mechanics

Prevent body stress and injury with proper technique.

Objectives:

- Demonstrate good body mechanics
- Demonstrate good lifting techniques
- Explain ambulatory procedures
- Explain the importance of positioning
- Identify proper positioning
- Demonstrate how to move residents in bed
- Demonstrate how to transfer residents

Need-to-Know Words:
- body mechanics
- ambulate
- lifting
- positioning
- alignment
- transfer
- contractures
- pressure ulcers
- friction
- moving
- drawsheet
- gurney

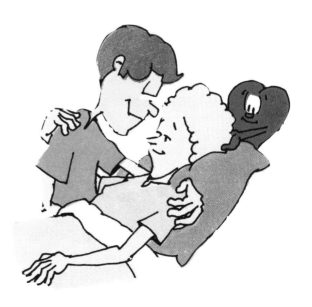

Part 1 Lifting

Good lifting techniques help prevent injuries.

Lifting Guidelines

- Evaluate the situation.
- Get help if needed.
- Prepare the area for a safe move.
- Lift only when necessary; push, pull, or roll whenever appropriate.
- Keep your back straight.
- Position your feet apart, one slightly ahead of the other.
- Stand close to the object you are lifting.
- Do not twist your back.
- Do not bend at the waist.
- Bend your knees and lift with your leg muscles.

1. Explain to the resident what you are going to do, and provide privacy as necessary.
2. Prepare the area for the move and for safe lifting.
3. Wash your hands before and after lifting or moving anyone.
4. If the resident is able, explain how he or she can help with the move.
5. Check your stance. Feet should be shoulder width apart, knees slightly bent, pointing in the direction of the move. Position your body in a straight line; do not twist or bend.
6. Hold the person (or object) you are lifting close to you, without reaching or stretching.
7. Keep your back straight, bend at the knees, and use your legs to lift.
8. When lifting with a team, count "1, 2, 3, LIFT," and make sure everyone lifts together smoothly.
8. Stop if any team member is not ready or if the load shifts.
9. After the move, position the resident safely and comfortably.
10. Always place the call signal within easy reach of the resident when applicable.

Some residents cannot or should not move themselves. They need your help. Moving residents is a major cause of accidents and injuries in the healthcare profession. Using good body mechanics helps protect you and the resident from injury.

Body mechanics are how you stand, move, and position your body. Positioning your body—back, hips, and feet—in a straight line will prevent injury, and keep you from tiring quickly.

Always check the care plan before you begin any move. Make sure you can handle the load, if not, ask for assistance. Never try to lift too much by yourself. Consider safety first and foremost.

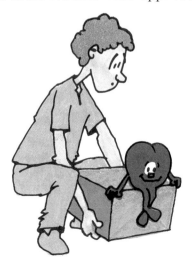

Part 2 — Ambulating

The ability to move from place to place promotes wellness.

Residents who are physically able should be encouraged to ambulate (walk) whenever possible. Check the care plan for type and amount of activity that is allowed. Mobility increases circulation, excercises muscles and joints, aids digestion, and maintains bowel functioning.

Be aware of each resident's ability to walk. Check the care plan to determine whether the person can walk unassisted, needs supervision, uses an assistive device (e.g., cane, walker), or requires hands-on assistance at all times. Never rush residents, and offer encouragement for their efforts.

Be alert at all times to any safety hazards, and observe each resident carefully for loss of balance or fatigue. Encourage residents to wear nonslip footwear and to use handrails.

For a resident who needs minimal assistance, walk alongside. Support the resident's bent arm (next to you) with your far hand. Place your near hand under the resident's armpit (on the side farthest from you).

A resident who is unsteady may need help to stand. Before assisting, tell the resident how to help, and arrange a signal (e.g., "1, 2, 3, stand"). Place a gait belt securely around the person. With shoes on, the person places feet flat on the floor. Facing the person, grasp both sides of the gait belt, and position yourself securely while you help the person stand.

After the person is stable, assist with walking. Keep one hand firmly on the belt, walking slightly behind and to one side.

Be alert to any sudden loss of balance. If a person starts to fall, do not try to stop the fall. Stopping the fall is likely to cause injury. Instead, sidestep and bend your knees to slowly ease the person to the floor. Stay with the person and call for help. Do not move the person until the nurse approves the move.

Part 3 — Positioning

Frequent repositioning helps prevent serious health problems.

Positioning is placement of the body for lying or sitting. Proper positioning and good body alignment add to a person's comfort. Staying in one position for too long can cause serious health problems. Aging skin is fragile; be gentle whenever you move or position someone.

Proper positioning includes the following benefits:

- promoting good circulation
- increasing comfort and well-being
- preventing joint deformities and contractures (shortening, tightening)
- preventing loss of muscle tone
- preventing edema (swelling)
- preventing pressure ulcers

Some residents cannot or should not move themselves. They need to be repositioned every hour or two. Certain positions may be restricted for some residents. Always check each care plan for any restrictions and frequency for positioning.

Before positioning a resident, explain what you are going to do, and provide privacy as needed. Ask the resident to help with the move if he or she is able. Assess the move. If you cannot handle the move alone, get help before you begin.

Move the person gently to a comfortable position with correct body alignment and support that minimizes pressure. Correctly position any nonfunctional limbs. Use rolled towels and pillows to cushion and support the body.

Pressure Ulcers

A pressure ulcer (alco called a decubitus ulcer, or pressure sore) is a serious skin problem related to inactivity. These wounds are painful, treatment is difficult, and complications can be very serious. Prevention depends on quality nursing care, frequent repositioning, and careful observation. Additional ways to help prevent pressure ulcers include the use of special pressure reducing beds, low air-loss alternating pressure mattresses, pressure relieving pads, cushions, and wedges.

Signs of pressure may indicate that the resident needs to be repositioned more often. Watch for irregularities such as pale, pinkish-red, or darkened skin color at pressure points. (See page 60.) Report your observations if the color does not return to normal after pressure is relieved.

Bed Positioning

Positioning requires proper body alignment and changing positions frequently. Check the care plan for any restrictions. Common positions for people who are confined to their beds are lateral, supine, Sims', prone, and Fowler's. Always position the resident so that alignment is good and the spine is straight. To check alignment, stand at the foot of the bed to see whether the resident's hip, shoulder, and ear are in a straight line. (Stand at the toes to see the nose.)

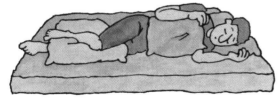

Lateral (lying on side)

Support the head, upper leg, and thigh with pillows. Place a pillow firmly against the back.

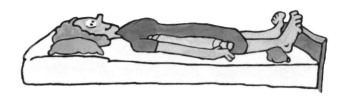

Supine (lying on back)

Support the feet at a right angle using a footboard or other device. Use a small pillow for the head. Prevent hip rotation by placing a trochanter roll (rolled up towel or small blanket) firmly against the hip. A small pillow at the ankles helps prevent pressure ulcers.

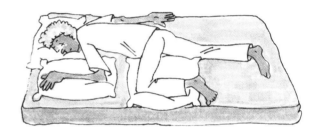

Sims' Position

Shoulders are nearly prone, and hips are in a side-lying position. Top leg is sharply flexed upward, and the lower arm is behind the resident. Use pillows to support the head, shoulder, flexed leg, and upper arm.

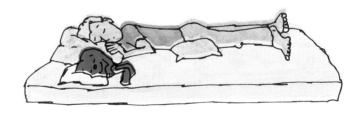

Prone (lying on stomach)

Always check with the nurse before putting a resident in this position (a weak person could suffocate). Turn the head to one side. Place a small pillow under the thighs to reduce strain on the back.

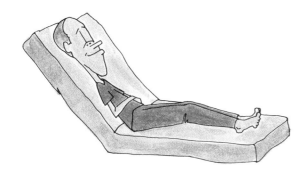

Fowler's Position

(sitting at 45-90 degree angle)

Semi-Fowler

(sitting at 30 degree angle with knees slightly bent)

Align head, trunk, and legs. Support the head and shoulders for easy breathing.

Chair Positioning

Residents who are able to get out of bed may choose to sit in chairs, and they may need your help. Always check each resident's care plan for any restrictions. Specific restrictions may apply because certain positions are harmful for the resident.

Before you begin the move, always check for safety hazards and determine whether you need someone to assist you. Safety is critical whenever you move or position a resident. Encourage the resident to help as much as possible. Place a gait belt securely around the person. Stand in front of him or her to assist with standing, and position yourself securely. Remember to use good body mechanics.

Follow these steps for chair positioning.

1. Slowly lower the person into the chair, as far back as possible, with hips pressing against the back of the chair.

2. Place feet so they are resting comfortably on the floor or on a footrest.

3. Position the back of the knees slightly beyond the edge of the chair to avoid any pressure.

4. If necessary, support the lower back with a pillow.

5. Support arms and hands with armrests or pillows.

6. Correct any slumping.

    · If the resident slumps sideways, place a pillow on that side for support and to straighten the spine.

    · If the resident slumps forward, align the spine by propping pillows on each side or in front.

    · A wedge pillow may be helpful to keep the resident sitting back in the chair.

7. Check the resident frequently for comfort and proper positioning.

Position the resident with the spine aligned (in a straight line) and the head erect. Keep the spine straight by using pillows on either side to prevent leaning. Some residents need body-support devices to maintain proper positioning while sitting. Use chair cushions, rolled towels, and skin-protection devices as needed. Poor positioning or sitting in one position for long periods of time can cause serious problems.

For any device that restrains movement and cannot be easily removed by the resident, a doctor's order is required. Examples of restraints are seatbelts, side rails, and position-change alarms. Be sure you know how to use/apply devices correctly. If not, ask your supervisor. Incorrect use of a device can cause serious injuries. Always follow the care plan, doctor's orders, and facility policies very carefully.

Minimize any pressure, and make sure circulation is good at all times. For residents at risk of pressure ulcers, use special pressure-reduction devices (e.g., therapeutic foam, air pads). Always consider the resident's comfort, function, and well-being. Check on residents often, and reposition frequently (every two hours or less).

Wheelchair Positioning

Ensure your own safety by using good body mechanics whenever you lift, move, or position residents. Applying good body mechanics helps prevent injury and is safer for both you and the residents.

Follow these steps to move a resident into a wheelchair. Then procedures are the same as chair positioning. (See page 31.)

1. Lock the wheels, and turn the footrests out of the way.

2. If needed, place a transfer (gait) belt around the resident's waist. Grasp the transfer belt at each side to assist with the move.

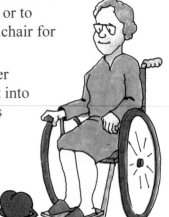

3. Ask the resident to place both hands on your waist or to hold on to the wheelchair for support.

4. Use the pivot transfer to move the resident into the chair. (See pages 34-35.)

5. Position the footrests and the resident's feet.

6. Ensure the resident's safety and comfort.

Part 4	Moving

Check the care plan for any restrictions before moving a resident.

People who are unable to move themselves need your help. Before moving anyone, check the care plan and assess the situation. If you need assistance, get help before you begin the move. Whenever possible work with a partner. Communicate your intentions clearly. (Example: "On the count of three, let's move the resident toward the headboard.")

When you move a resident, prevent friction (rubbing one surface against another). Sliding causes friction, so roll or lift the person rather than sliding. Friction is painful and can damage the skin.

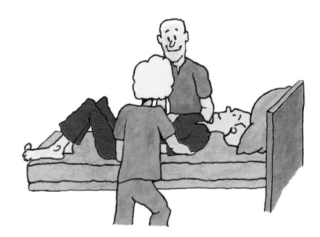

Moving Guidelines

Whenever you move a resident, follow these general guidelines (unless otherwise noted in the care plan).

1. Check identification to be sure you have the right person.

2. Explain what you are going to do, and provide privacy.

3. Wash your hands before and after moving a resident.

4. Lock all wheels (bed, wheelchair).

5. Adjust the bed so it is flat and at a level for good body mechanics.

6. Encourage the resident to help as much as possible.

7. Use good body mechanics, bending at the knees with your back straight.

8. After the move, position the resident, and place the call signal within easy reach.

To move a resident up in bed, get help if needed or secure the side rail on the far side (if allowed*). Put a pillow against the headboard to prevent injury. Place one arm under the resident's shoulders and the other arm under the thighs. If able, ask the resident to put feet flat on the bed and bend at the knees. On the count of three, have the resident push with the feet while you lift toward the head of the bed.

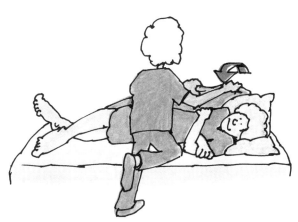

To turn a resident toward you, cross the person's arms over the chest. Place your arms at the shoulder and hip on the far side. Gently draw the side that is away from you toward you (crossing the far leg over the near leg), rolling the body as one unit. Position the person, aligning the legs with the upper body, and place a pillow at the back for support.

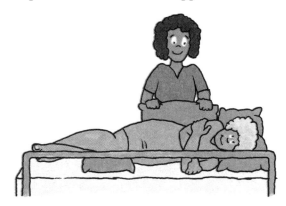

To turn a resident away from you, raise the rail on the far side (if allowed*). Cross the person's arms over the chest. Gently roll the person — as one unit — toward the raised rail (cross the near leg over the far leg). Position, align, and place pillows for support. Lower the side rail.

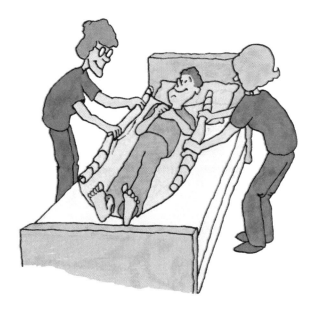

To move a resident with a drawsheet (folded sheet or blanket), you need assistance. A drawsheet is used to move someone who cannot help or is very fragile. Place a drawsheet under the resident from shoulders to mid-thigh, with six inches or more on both sides to hold onto. Grip the sheet firmly at the shoulders and hips. On the count of three, lift the person smoothly to the desired position.

If the move is from a bed to gurney (stretcher), secure the gurney next to the bed and lock the wheels on both devices. As soon as the person is on the gurney, attach safety straps and stay with the person.

*Beds are equipped with side rails that can be raised to keep residents safe. However, a raised side rail is classified as a restraint. Always follow the care plan and facility policy for using side rails.

Log rolling is a two-person move for a resident with spinal injuries who must be moved without changing body alignment. The torso, hips, and legs must be moved as one unit in straight alignment. Position the resident's arm across the chest, and place a pillow or wedge between the legs. Use a pillow under the head and also a small pillow at the mid-section if needed to maintain alignment.

With your hands on the far shoulder and hip, you and your partner gently roll the person toward you onto his or her side, turning the body as one unit (like rolling a log). Align and position the resident, with support at the back.

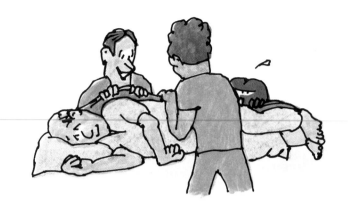

Part 5 — Transferring

Encourage the resident to help with the transfer as much as possible.

Some residents need help when they transfer (move) from one place to another (e.g., from bed to chair). NAs transfer residents many times a day. Whenever residents can assist with transfers, encourage their help. Take every precaution to ensure safety and to prevent injuries to yourself or residents. Follow each resident's care plan, and use the best transfer techniques based on individual needs.

Always assess the situation. Ask for assistance if you need it. Plan ahead for any equipment you may need, and clear the pathway for the transfer.

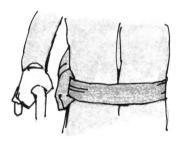

A transfer (gait) belt provides a grip for the NA and adds to the resident's safety during transfers.

Examples of transfers include the following:

- bed to wheelchair and wheelchair to bed
- bed to toilet or commode and return to bed
- wheelchair to toilet and toilet to wheelchair
- wheelchair to tub or shower and return to wheelchair

Always use good body mechanics to prevent injuries to yourself and others.

The pivot transfer is used for residents who are hemiplegic (paralyzed on one side). Follow these steps to move the resident from bed to chair.

1. Check identification to be sure you have the right person.

2. Explain what you are going to do, and provide privacy.

3. Keep transfer sites close together, equalizing heights as much as possible.

4. Lock all wheels (bed, wheelchair).

5. Put the bed at its lowest position with the head raised to a sitting position.

6. Help the resident to a sitting position with feet flat on the floor.

7. Stay with the resident, and allow time to gain balance if needed.

8. Assist with robe and nonslip footwear, and apply a transfer belt.

9. Position the chair on the resident's strong side, at the head of the bed, wheels locked, and footrests folded or removed.

10. Stand in front of the resident, bracing your legs and grasping the transfer belt on both sides.

11. Lifting with your legs (not your back), have the resident lean toward the strong side while you support the weak side.

12. Slowly and smoothly turn the resident (without twisting) to the front of the wheelchair.

13. Gently lower the person into the chair, with hips against the back of the chair.

14. Remove the belt, and position with good alignment (with feet on footrests).

To transfer the resident back into bed, reverse the procedure. Place the call signal within easy reach.

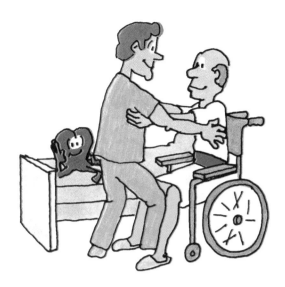

Assistive Transfer
(resident is able to help)

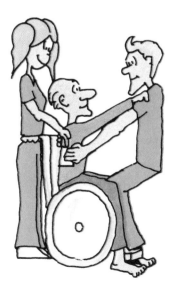

Passive Transfer
(resident is unable to help; at least two people are needed for the transfer)

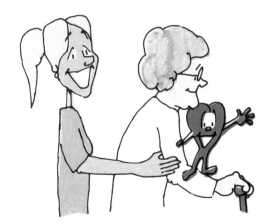

Active Transfer
(resident moves with minimal help)

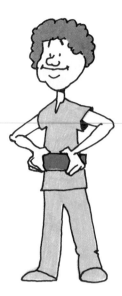

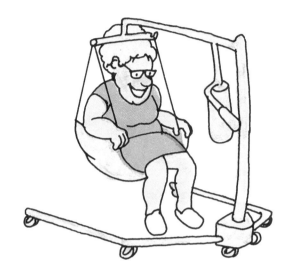

The **transfer belt** is placed around the resident's waist to provide a grip for the NA in transferring. It is used when transferring a semi-helpless or helpless resident. The belt is called a **gait belt** when used to assist in walking.

The **patient lift** (hydraulic or battery powered) is used for non-weight bearing residents. Always have assistance when operating the lift. Make sure you understand the operation. Ask your supervisor for help if you have any doubt. The lift is never used to transport a resident.

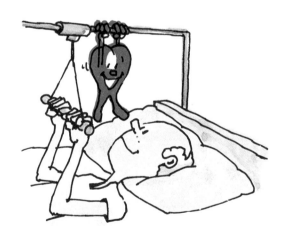

Follow procedures at the facility where you work for using all lifting and positioning equipment. Do not use any equipment without thorough training. Know your limitations, and be sure that adequate staff is available to assist and ensure safety.

The **trapeze bar** is a swinging bar hanging over the bed from a metal frame. The resident grasps the bar with both hands and lifts the torso (top of body) off the bed. The trapeze may be used for moving a resident up in bed, turning in bed, and to strengthen the arm muscles.

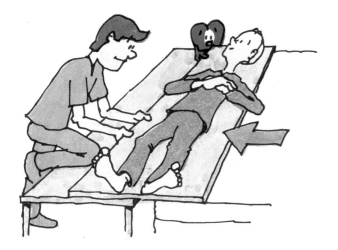

The **transfer board** keeps the back straight during transfer of a helpless patient. The transfer board is used when there is danger of spinal injury. Use only when both surfaces are at the same level.

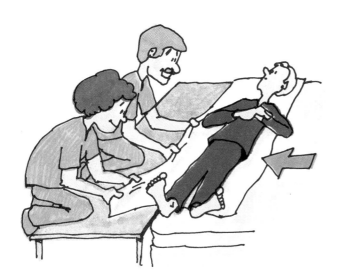

The **drawsheet** is used to transfer residents when there is no danger of back injury. For helpless residents, at least two NAs are required for the transfer. Use only when both surfaces are at the same level.

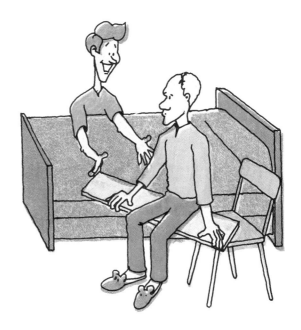

The **slide board** is a small board placed between the bed and a chair or wheelchair. The resident sits on the board and is helped to slide across the board into the desired position. The slide board is used when there is no danger of spinal injury. Use only when both surfaces are at similar levels.

Summary

Protect yourself and the residents from injuries by always using good body mechanics. Check each resident's care plan for any restrictions, and promote maximum independence. Encourage walking for residents who are able, and assist as needed. Reposition residents often to prevent complications. Ensure everyone's safety and well-being whenever you lift, move, or position anyone.

Review

1. What are good body mechanics, and why are they important for the NA?

5. Why is frequent repositioning important?

2. Describe correct lifting procedures.

6. What are two major problems of inactivity?

3. Explain three or more benefits of walking.

7. How do you know when to reposition a resident?

4. If a person starts to fall while walking, what should you do?

8. What is a transfer belt, and when should it be used?

Module 5

Preventing/ Controlling Infection

Guard against possible infection at all times.

Objectives:

- Describe ways to prevent infection
- Practice precautions
- Identify procedures for medical asepsis
- Explain the importance of hand washing
- Demonstrate proper hand-washing procedures
- Describe sterilizing and disinfecting
- Discuss the need for protective barriers
- Demonstrate proper use of gloves
- Describe isolation procedures
- Explain how to control HBV
- Identify ways to prevent HIV/AIDS

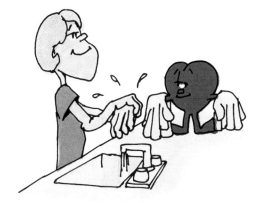

Need-to-Know Words:

- infection prevention
- infection control
- medical asepsis
- immune system
- susceptible
- precautions
- microorganisms
- pathogens
- contaminated
- sterilizing
- disinfecting
- isolation
- protective barriers
- transmit

Part 1	Preventing Infection

Preventing problems is easier than curing them.

Infection prevention and control are critical concerns for healthcare workers. Control measures apply to everything from colds and flu to life-threatening diseases.

Infection is spread by microorganisms (living organisms that can be seen only with a microscope). Microorganisms are everywhere—in the air, on the skin, in food and beverages, and on everything you touch. There are two types of microorganisms—pathogenic (harmful) and nonpathogenic (harmless). Microorganisms that cause disease are bacteria (e.g., staph or strep), virus, and fungus.

Infection spreads through contact with a contaminated person or object. Sneezing, coughing, and touching can spread germs.

Pathogens usually enter the body through broken or damaged skin, or through the mucous membranes of the eyes, nose, or mouth. Stop infection from spreading by being aware of how infection spreads.

The "chain of infection" has six links. Interrupting any of the links, stops infection from spreading. Following is a brief description of the chain of infection.

Infectious Agent	Carrier
pathogen	organism that produces disease
reservoir	where organisms grow and reproduce; often moist and warm
portal of exit	how germs get out of the reservoir (e.g., body fluid)
transmission	how germs spread from source to person
portal of entry	how germs get inside a new host (e.g., mouth, nose, eyes, cuts)
susceptible host	person lacking resistance to particular infection

Breaking any link breaks the chain. The weakest link is transmission. Most efforts to stop infection from spreading are aimed at eliminating the way germs are transmitted (e.g., washing hands, using personal protective equipment, disinfecting).

The immune system is the body's natural defense against infection. The system sometimes fails when powerful pathogens are present. Stress, poor nutrition, and lack of sleep tend to weaken resistance to disease.

Help residents recognize signs and symptoms of infection, and ask them to tell you whenever there is a problem. Encourage them to use tissues and cover their mouths when they cough or sneeze.

Following are examples of signs and symptoms that could indicate infection:

- fever or chills
- red or hot skin
- nausea or vomiting
- lack of appetite
- change in behavior

- restlessness
- pain
- swelling
- discharge or drainage
- diarrhea

Promptly report any changes in a resident's condition. Early detection can prevent infection from spreading.

Do Not Spread Infection!

- If you feel ill, (e.g., fever, nausea, vomiting, diarrhea, sore throat, coughing or sneezing), check with your supervisor before reporting for work.
- Cover any cuts or open sores with a fresh bandage before reporting for work.

Part 2 — Practicing Medical Asepsis

The single most important measure for infection prevention/control is hand washing.

The spread of infection is greatly reduced by medical asepsis (procedures to decrease pathogens). Always follow procedures to protect yourself and others from infection. Medical asepsis includes the following:

- hand washing
- clean surroundings
- personal hygiene
- precautions

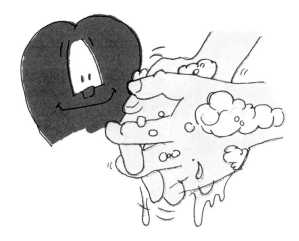

WASH YOUR HANDS!

- Before and after your work shift
- Before and after breaks and meals
- Before and after each resident contact
- After using the toilet
- After coughing, sneezing, blowing your nose
- After handling bedpans, feces, specimens, used bandages and dressings
- After handling soiled linen or a resident's personal belongings
- Before and after wearing disposable gloves

---

4. Clean your fingernails by rubbing soapy fingertips against the palm of the opposite hand. (Keep nails short.)

5. Rinse well with warm running water (hands lower than your elbows and fingertips down).

6. Pat dry thoroughly with a clean paper towel, and dispose of the towel.

7. Use a clean, dry paper towel to turn off the water, and dispose of the towel.

Hand washing is the single most important way to prevent/control the spread of infection.

Prevent the spread of infection by taking time to wash your hands thoroughly, following these step-by-step procedures.

1. Assemble all equipment before you begin.
   - soap
   - paper towels
   - wastebasket

2. Run water until warm, and completely wet your hands and wrists.

3. Apply soap, and lather vigorously — hands, wrists, fingers — for at least 20 seconds.

Germs are commonly found in moist and warm areas. Whenever you wash your hands, avoid touching the sink or faucets at any time. Use a clean paper towel to turn on the water. Then use another clean towel to turn off the water. Do not crumple the towel (to avoid any contact with an infected area of the towel).

Keep your clothing away from the sink, wastebasket, and faucets, and do not touch them with your clean hands. Use facility-approved hand lotion to prevent chapping from frequent hand washing.

Clean Surroundings

You can prevent infection from spreading by providing residents with clean surroundings. Sterilization, disinfection, and proper linen handling are important methods for controlling infection. Always place used equipment and supplies in the designated areas.

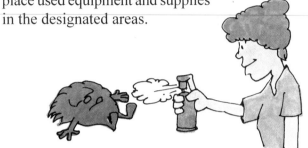

Sterilizing kills all bacteria. Unless all bacteria are dead, an object is not sterile. A sterile object becomes contaminated when exposed to air or other objects. Diagnostic equipment and metal bedpans are most commonly sterilized by autoclaving (an intense heat process).

Disinfecting requires chemicals that kill most of the bacteria. Those that are not killed are slowed in their growth. Reusable plastic bedpans, trays, and equipment are sanitized (washed in a bacterial cleanser), dried, and stored in clean bags.

Bed Linen

Use precautions when handling bed linen. Soiled linen can transfer germs.

Follow these guidelines.

- Wash your hands before handling clean linen.

- Avoid touching linen with your clothing.

- Bring into the room only the linen to be used at that time.

- Keep clean and dirty linen separated; clean linen carts should be six feet or more from soiled linen hampers.

- Wear gloves to handle linen that is soiled with blood or body fluids.

- Always roll soiled linen away from you, and avoid shaking or fluffing the linen.

- Keep all linen (clean and soiled) off the floor.

- Place soiled linen in covered hampers or bags immediately to prevent the spread of infection and to control odors.

- Always wash your hands after handling soiled linen.

Part 3   **Using Precautions**

Treat everyone with care and caution.

Precautions establish safe practices to protect healthcare workers. Universal Precautions were established in 1988 to prevent the spread of deadly blood-borne pathogens. Standard Precautions, developed in 1996, promote the use of personal protective equipment (e.g., gloves, gowns, masks, eyewear) for contact with *all* body fluids (except sweat).

Infected people often have no symptoms and may not know they are infected, Therefore, consider yourself at risk from everyone. Follow infection-control practices and procedures at the facility where you work. Precautions reduce the risk of spreading germs from person to person.

Provide quality care for all residents, and use precautions with each person, all used needles, and all body fluids.

> Assume all blood, body fluids, and needles are potentially infectious. Gloves must be worn at all times when handling these materials. Always wash your hands before and after wearing gloves.

Personal Protective Equipment

Gloves, gowns, aprons, masks, and protective eyewear are necessary whenever you might be exposed to blood or body fluids, non-intact skin, and mucous membranes (mouth, nose, eyes, genital area). Personal protective equipment (PPE) is a barrier between you and possible sources of infection.

Gloves reduce the risk of spreading infection. Always wear disposable gloves whenever you have contact with any of the following:

- bleeding or open wounds (skin rashes, broken skin, pressure ulcers)
- other body fluids, including blood
- soiled linen

Follow these guidelines for using gloves:

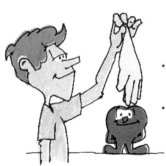

- Check for cracks, punctures, tears, or discoloration, and discard if damaged.
- Check for proper fit; avoid wrinkles.
- Wash your hands before putting on gloves.
- Pull gloves over gown cuffs if a gown is worn.

Change gloves whenever they become soiled to avoid spreading infection from one part of the body to another. Dispose of gloves after each resident contact.

To remove gloves, use one gloved hand to grasp the other glove near the wrist and peel off the glove, pulling it inside-out. Hold it in the gloved hand. Slide fingers from the bare hand under the wrist of the other glove, peel off, creating a bag for both gloves. Dispose in the designated bin for infectious waste, and wash your hands.

Face masks may be required to protect residents, workers, and visitors from infection caused by airborne pathogens or exposure to blood and body fluids. Wash your hands before touching the mask. Pick up the mask by the straps, and avoid touching the part that covers your nose and mouth.

Masks should be changed frequently and anytime they become damp or wet. Dispose of used masks immediately in the appropriate waste container, and wash your hands.

Gowns are effective barriers to infection whenever you have direct contact with infectious material or body fluids. Roll your sleeves above your elbows, and wash your hands before putting on a gown.

Before removing the gown, remove and dispose of the gloves. Pull the gown away from neck and shoulders. Holding the gown away from you, turn it inward, keeping it inside out. Place the gown in the appropriate container, and wash your hands.

Isolation

Residents with highly transmissible diseases are sometimes isolated (set apart) to protect others from infection. In addition to using Standard Precautions, you may be instructed to follow **transmission-based precautions**—contact, droplet, and airborne precautions—that vary according to the specific disease and how the pathogens are transmitted. Sometimes isolation is ordered for residents who cannot fight infection due to age, illness, or medications.

Doctors order isolation precautions. Instructions are generally posted on the door of isolation rooms. The instructions may direct all visitors to report to the nurses' station before entering the room. Or, the signs may specify that personal protective equipment — gowns, masks, and gloves — is required each time anyone enters the room.

All basic supplies and equipment for the care of the isolated resident should be stored in the room. Gather any additional equipment before you put on isolation gear to enter the room.

It is not uncommon for isolated residents to be lonely and depressed. The NA can help ease depression in a variety of ways. Following are examples.

- Check on the person often, and answer the call signal promptly.
- Spend time with the resident.
- Provide access to television, radio, magazines, puzzles and other amusements.
- Tell the resident when you will be back, and be prompt; let the resident know if you are delayed.
- Be cautious of what you say outside the room; the resident may hear you.
- Help the resident, family, and visitors be comfortable and confident with the isolation procedures.

Other Precautions

Use extreme caution with needles and infectious waste. Be aware of how infection is spread, and use personal protective equipment to protect yourself and others from infection.

Following are additional precautions and safety measures.

- Handle all needles very carefully, and dispose of them in designated biohazard containers.
- Be aware that gloves will not protect you from being stuck by a needle. If you stick yourself with a used needle, wash the punctured area immediately with hot, soapy water. Then tell your supervisor.
- Be very careful whenever you handle infectious waste. Follow the facility's guidelines for handling waste.
- Report all broken skin contact, mucous membrane contact, and puncture wounds.
- Change gloves each time you go from one resident to another.
- Wear a mask, gown, gloves, and protective eyewear for any procedures that could involve blood or body fluid splashing.
- If you are pregnant and working in a high-risk area, get medical counseling.

Part 4	**Controlling Hepatitis B Virus (HBV)**

Vaccination can prevent Hepatitis B infection.

Hepatitis B Virus (HBV) is a viral infection of the liver. The disease causes fatigue, mild fever, muscle and joint pain, nausea, vomiting, and loss of appetite. There is no known cure for HBV at this time.

HBV usually spreads through contact with infected blood, blood products, body fluids, or anywhere blood is present.

Following are examples of how the virus spreads:

- intimate sexual contact
- damaged skin (e.g., cuts, rashes)
- puncture wounds from contaminated needles or sharp objects
- mucous membranes (eyes, nose, mouth)

A blood test is the only way to find out if a person is infected. Get a blood test. If you are not infected, consider being vaccinated to protect yourself.

Part 5 — Preventing HIV/AIDS

Always use precautions with all body fluids, especially blood.

AIDS (Acquired Immune Deficiency Syndrome) is a life-threatening condition caused by a virus known as HIV (Human Immunodeficiency Virus). The virus cripples the immune system, the body's natural defense against disease. By destroying cells, HIV interferes with the ability to fight off viruses, bacteria, and fungi. The term AIDS refers to the later stages of HIV infection.

There is no cure and no vaccine at this time for HIV/AIDS. The best defense is preventive education. It is important to understand how the disease spreads and how to protect yourself and others.

You will not get AIDS from casual contact. The disease is transmitted when contaminated (infected) fluid enters the bloodstream. Of these fluids, blood is the most common concern for healthcare workers.

Following are ways the virus enters the body:

- intimate sexual contact
- transfusions with infected blood
- puncture wounds from infected needles or broken glass
- cuts or open sores
- mucous membranes (nose, mouth, eyes)
- use of infected hypodermic needles
- infected mothers to their unborn babies

When people are infected with HIV, they are carriers for life. People may not know they are infected. Some carriers never show symptoms, but they can still transmit HIV to others.

Symptoms vary from person to person. In the early stages, people with HIV usually look and feel healthy. Early symptoms are often similar to common illnesses—coughing, fever, swollen glands, diarrhea. The symptoms go away, but the HIV remains in the body. Advanced symptoms may develop five to fourteen years later.

AIDS victims are susceptible to diseases the body would normally resist. As the disease progresses, the immune system is unable to fight infection. Treatment can increase the length of survival, but there is no cure.

Always use precautions to protect yourself and others from infection. Treat all blood and body fluids as contaminated. Wear gloves whenever you have contact with body fluids or soiled articles. Wash your hands with soap and water after any contact with blood, even if gloves are worn. Use the same precautions with vaginal secretions and semen.

Pour all liquid waste containing blood down the toilet. Avoid splashing on yourself. Put the toilet lid down, and flush. Also flush tissues and other flushable items with blood or body fluids on them. Use a disposal bag for paper towels, wound dressings, sanitary pads, and other solid waste. Close the bag securely. Follow disposal regulations for the facility where you work.

Summary

Protect yourself, residents, co-workers, and visitors from infection by using precautions. The best defense is understanding how infection spreads and using preventive measures. Thorough hand washing is the single most important preventive measure for infection control. Other important measures include clean surroundings, personal protective equipment, and isolation precautions. Always protect residents from infection, provide quality care, and treat all body fluids and needles as potentially infectious.

Review

1. What are Universal and Standard Precautions?

2. How can you protect yourself from infection?

3. Describe how infection spreads.

4. Explain isolation procedures.

5. Give five or more examples of when you must wash your hands.

6. Give three or more examples of when to wear gloves.

7. Identify three or more ways that HBV infection is spread.

8. How is HIV/AIDS transmitted?

Module 6

Weighing and Measuring

Accuracy is important in everything you do.

Objectives:

- Demonstrate procedures for weighing residents
- Demonstrate procedures for measuring residents
- Identify fluid measurements

Need-to-Know Words:

- measurement
- metric system
- centimeter
- kilogram
- height
- weight
- convert

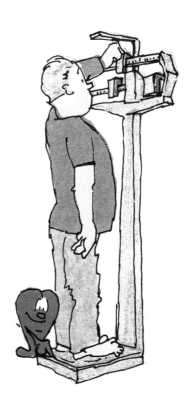

Part 1 — Weighing and Measuring

Changes in weight and height may indicate health problems.

Residents are weighed and measured when they are admitted to the facility and periodically thereafter. Accuracy is important. Changes may indicate health problems. Learn to use the scales in your facility safely and correctly.

The most commonly used equipment for weighing and measuring is the standing balance scale with a measuring rod. For residents who cannot stand, there are bed, wheelchair, and mechanical-lift scales.

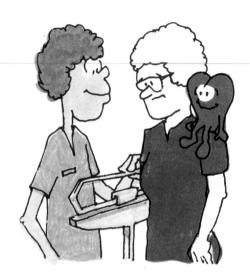

Guidelines for Weighing

- Weigh at the same time of day.
- Wear the same weight of clothing.
- Weigh with an empty bladder.

Weighing (Standing balance scale)

The resident needs to wear shoes to walk to/from the scale. (Follow facility policy regarding footwear during weighing.) Following are the steps to weigh on a standing balance scale.

1. Place both weights at zero.

2. Stand next to the scale, and assist the resident onto the center of the scale.

3. Slide the bottom weight until the balance drops, and move the weight back one slot. (Make sure the resident is not holding onto you or the scale.)

4. Slide the top weight until the balance centers.

5. Determine the resident's weight by adding the numbers shown at both weights.

6. Assist the person off the scale, or proceed with height measurement.

7. Chart the weight, and report any significant changes.

Weight Measurements

Healthcare facilities often use the metric system for measurements. Nursing Assistants should have basic understanding of the metric system. Most facilities have charts available to help convert (change) measurements.

Weight is measured in pounds and ounces or in kilograms. Following are examples of weight measurements:

lb = pound	oz = ounce
kg = kilogram	

8 oz = 1/2 lb	16 oz = 1 lb
1 lb = .45 kg	2.2 lb = 1 kg
100 lb = 45.36 kg	1 stone = 14 lb (British)

Height Measurements

The best time to measure height is when the resident is on the scale for weighing. Follow these steps for measuring on a standing balance scale.

1. Assist the resident to turn towards you and to stand straight.

2. Place the measuring rod level against the top of the resident's head.

3. Read the resident's height.

4. Help the resident off the scale before recording height.

5. Chart the height, and report any changes.

Height is measured in feet and inches or in centimeters. One centimeter equals .39 inches. Following are examples of height measurements:

in or " = inch
ft or ' = foot
mm = millimeter
cm = centimeter
m = meter

12 in = 1 foot
3 ft = 1 yard
1 m = 3.28 feet

Residents who are confined to their beds need to be weighed and measured in bed. Before using a bed scale, be sure you know how to use the equipment correctly and safely. Follow the manufacturer's instructions and the facility's procedures.

Use a tape measure for measuring a resident in bed. With the resident lying straight, make marks at the top of the head and the bottom of the feet. Measure the distance between the two marks, and record the resident's height.

Fluid Measurements

You may be required to measure the exact amount of fluid intake and output for some residents and to record the fluid in cubic centimeters (cc) or milliliters (mL).

Following are examples of fluid measurements:

cc = cubic centimeter
mL = milliliter
oz = ounce

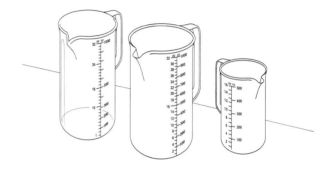

1 cc = 1 mL
30 cc = 1 ounce
5 cc = 1 teaspoon
32 ounces = 1 quart
33.8 ounces = 1 liter

Many containers used in care facilities are marked with both ounces and cubic centimeters. Most facilities provide conversion charts for fluid measurements and the capacity of containers used in the facility. To convert ounces to centimeters, simply multiply the number of ounces by 30. For example, 16 ounces (one pint) multiplied by 30 equals 480 cubic centimeters.

Summary

Learn to use equipment safely and correctly for weighing and measuring residents. Accuracy is critical; changes in measurements may indicate health problems. If you are unsure about safe and accurate procedures, ask your supervisor for help.

Review

1. Explain why accuracy is important for weighing and measuring.

_____

_____

_____

_____

2. Describe steps for weighing a resident with a standing balance scale.

_____

_____

_____

_____

3. List three units for measuring weight.

_____

_____

_____

_____

4. Describe steps for measuring height of a resident with a standing balance scale.

_____

_____

_____

_____

5. List three units for measuring height.

_____

_____

_____

_____

6. List three units for measuring fluids.

_____

_____

_____

_____

7. Explain how to measure a resident in bed.

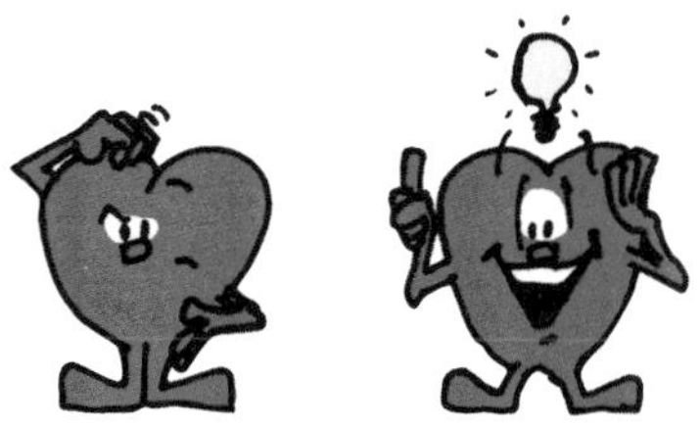

_____

_____

_____

_____

Module 7

Providing Basic Care

Good skills earn the respect of residents and co-workers.

Objectives:

- Describe personal hygiene
- Identify three methods of bathing
- Explain procedures for foot and nail care
- Demonstrate procedures for oral hygiene
- Describe hair care
- Identify pressure points
- Demonstrate the use of bedpans
- Discuss bowel and bladder problems
- Explain effects of aging on digestion

Need-to-Know Words:

- timelines
- military time
- perineal care
- oral hygiene
- emesis basin
- NPO orders
- skin injury
- pressure points
- integumentary
- shearing
- mottled
- elimination
- impaction
- incontinence
- urinal
- fracture pan
- commode
- digestion

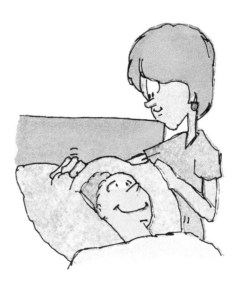

Part 1	**Promoting Personal Hygiene**

Cleanliness promotes good health, and looking good boosts morale.

The NA's daily routine includes many activities to keep the resident clean and comfortable. Personal hygiene (cleanliness) is important for maintaining health. Good grooming enhances self-esteem.

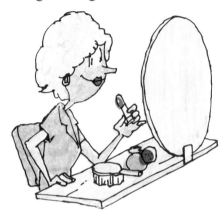

Some residents are able to maintain their own hygiene and appearance. Others may need your assistance. And some are completely dependent on you for care. Maintain adequate supplies and equipment for each resident's personal use.

Provide training in self-care, and encourage each resident to be as self-managing as possible. Offer support, encouragement, and assistance as needed. Provide care that is appropriate for each person's needs, preferences, and customs. Report any pain, discomfort, or changes in a resident's condition.

Follow care procedures at the facility where you work. Before providing personal care, always check each resident's care plan for any restrictions.

Sometimes residents need specific care at specified times, and meeting those timelines is important. Instructions may specify a.m. (midnight to noon) and p.m. (noon to midnight) or military time (based on a 24-hour clock). Military time begins at midnight with zero hour.

Following are examples of military time:

    00:05 = 12:05 a.m.   20:15 = 8:15 p.m.

*See Flash Cards for Time-Conversion Chart.

Bathing

Every morning (a.m.) and every evening (p.m.) residents are given care consisting of washing the face, back, armpits, and perineum. Always provide privacy.

Bathing provides more than cleanliness. Baths encourage exercise, stimulate circulation, prevent pressure ulcers, and promote relaxation. Baths give the NA an opportunity to spot problems such as infections or pressure ulcers. Encourage residents to wash themselves if they are able.

Perineal Care

Perineal care (or pericare) is cleansing of the genitalia and rectum. Pericare is given during the daily bath and after urinating or defecating. **Cleansing is always done from the front to the back** to prevent urinary tract infection.

1. Gather all equipment before you begin.
   - bath blanket
   - bed protector
   - washcloths
   - soap
   - wash basin
   - towels
   - warm water
   - gloves

2. Wash your hands, and put on gloves.

3. Explain what you are going to do, and provide privacy.

4. Place the bed protector under the resident's buttocks, and cover the resident with a bath blanket.

5. Make a washcloth into a mitt by folding it into thirds around your dominant hand – fold the top down and tuck it under the bottom edge. Making a mitt helps prevent the dangling ends of a washcloth from dripping water onto the resident.

6. Squeeze the mitt in warm soapy water. Separate the labia (female) with one hand and cleanse the area with the mitt, wipe from front to back, rinsing and changing location on the washcloth with each wipe. Clean the penis (male) from tip downward with gentle circular motions. Pull back the foreskin of the uncircumcised male to clean the area.

7. Use clean, warm water and a clean washcloth to rinse the area, and gently pat dry with a towel.

8. Help the resident to a side-lying position.

9. Apply soap to a clean washcloth, and wash the rectum area (front to back).

10. Rinse and pat dry the area thoroughly.

11. Dispose of used linen, bed protector, and supplies in designated areas, avoiding contact with yourself or your clothing.

12. Position the resident comfortably, and adjust bedding.

13. Remove gloves, and wash your hands.

14. Report anything unusual—odors, discharges, swelling, redness.

Bed Baths

Full or partial bed baths are necessary for non-ambulatory residents. Encourage the resident to help as much as possible.

1. Assemble all supplies before you begin:
   - washcloths
   - towels
   - soap
   - bath blanket
   - basin with warm water
   - clean gown
   - gloves

2. Wash your hands, and put on gloves.

3. Keep the resident covered as much as possible.

4. Provide privacy, and close doors and windows to prevent drafts.

5. Offer toileting, and assist as needed.

6. Adjust bed to a comfortable working height.

7. Remove the blankets, and place a bath blanket.

8. Remove the resident's gown, and use the bath blanket to cover the resident.

9. Fill the basin two-thirds full with warm water.

10. Help the resident move toward you.

11. Place a towel under the resident's farthest side to keep the bed dry.

12. Using a clean mitted washcloth, wet with clean water only. Wash the eyes from the inner to the outer corner; rinse the cloth after washing each eye.

13. Wash the resident's face, neck, and ears with soapy washcloth. Rinse and pat dry with towel.

14. Work from the head down, washing with long, circular motions; rinse, and pat dry.

15. Change the water frequently when it is soapy or cool.

16. If the resident is able, offer the washcloth for cleaning the perineal area.

17. Turn the resident to a side-lying position and place a towel on the bottom sheet by the resident's back.

18. Wash, rinse, and dry the backside.

19. Place a towel under the legs, and bend the knees to wash and dry the legs and feet.

20. Apply deodorant, and put on a clean gown.

21. Make the resident comfortable, and place the call light/signal within easy reach.

22. Empty the basin, and dispose of linen and supplies in designated areas.

23. Remove gloves, and wash your hands.

Safety Guidelines for Bathing

- Use extreme caution to prevent slips and falls.
- Test the water temperature, then have the resident test it.
- Always assist residents in and out of the tub or shower.
- Never leave residents alone while bathing.

Shower Bath

1. Assemble all supplies before the shower:
   - towel
   - soap
   - washcloth
   - clean gown or clothes
2. Use a shower chair for safety and comfort (so the resident does not have to stand for long periods).

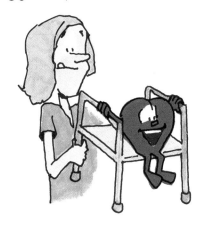

3. Check the water temperature before the resident enters the shower.
4. Assist the resident into the shower.
   - Steady an ambulatory resident with your arm.
   - For a resident in a wheelchair, wheels are locked during transfer to the shower chair.
5. Encourage self-care, and assist as needed with washing, rinsing, patting dry, and dressing.

Tub Baths

1. Assemble the same equipment as needed for a shower bath.
2. Fill the tub half full; test the water temperature, and ask the resident to test for comfort (generally 105°).

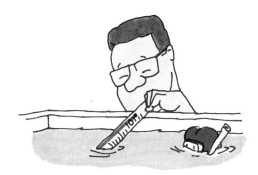

3. Place a rubber mat in the tub to prevent slipping (if the tub does not have safety strips).
4. If necessary, assist the resident into the tub.
5. Encourage self-care, and assist as needed with washing, rinsing, drying, and dressing.

Dressing

Encourage residents to dress and undress themselves if they are able. Assist only as needed, following these guidelines.

1. Help select appropriate clothing.
2. Prepare clothing by unbuttoning, unhooking, unzipping, and place the clothing on a chair in the order it will be used.
3. Provide privacy, and avoid overexposure.
4. Gently remove clothing, starting with the upper body first; do not force or overextend any joint.
5. If a resident has a weak side, remove clothing from the stronger side first; to put on clothing, dress the weaker side first.

6. Gently assist the resident to dress.

- Slacks: gather them at the leg, and guide the resident's foot through.
- Shirt or dress: gently pull the resident's hand through the sleeve.
- Pullovers: gently guide both arms into the sleeves and slide the garment over the resident's head.
- Elastic stockings: turn inside out to the heel area. With the person lying down, gently stretch stockings wrinkle-free over the foot, heel, and leg.

7. Adjust and fasten the clothing as needed.

8. Place dirty clothing in the appropriate hamper, and tidy the area.

9. Wash your hands.

Foot Care

Check the care plan thoroughly before giving foot care. Residents who are diabetic or have poor circulation require special care because they are at risk of infection. Avoid anything tight that might restrict circulation to the feet, ankles, or legs.

Examine feet daily. Notify your supervisor if there are red or irritated areas on the feet or if there are red or "hot" areas on the legs.

Bathe feet every day with soap and lukewarm water. Lift feet one at a time to wash them (including between the toes), while supporting the foot and ankle. Rinse well, and pat dry with a soft towel, taking care to dry between the toes. Apply lotion to top and bottom of both feet, and wipe away any excess. Tidy the area, and store equipment properly.

Following are additional guidelines for foot care.

- Put on clean socks every day.
- Alternate shoes daily to allow the worn pair to air.
- Check that shoes fit properly, do not restrict circulation, and are safe for walking.

- Check for blisters, sores, corns, infections, or swelling.
- Be aware that smoking reduces circulation to the feet.
- Report any foot problems promptly.

Nail Care

Always check with your supervisor before giving nail care. Only a licensed nurse is allowed to trim nails for some residents (e.g., people with diabetes). The resident's nails should be short, smooth, and clean.

For fingernail care, follow these steps.

1. Assemble all equipment before you begin:
   - nail file
   - orange sticks
   - emery board
   - clippers
   - basin with warm water
   - polish
   - tissues
   - lotion
   - towel

2. Wash your hands, and put on gloves.

3. Explain what you are going to do.

4. Soak nails in warm water (generally 105°).

5. As you dry the hands, gently push the cuticle back with the towel.

6. Feel each nail and file as needed.

7. Smooth and round fingernails with an emery board.

8. Carefully clean under each nail with an orange stick, and wipe the stick clean on a tissue before cleaning the next nail.

9. Apply hand lotion, and polish the nails if the resident desires.

10. Tidy the area, and dispose of supplies and equipment in designated areas.

11. Remove gloves, and wash your hands.

For toenail care (if approved), follow the same procedures as fingernails with these exceptions.

- Trim toenails straight across, and carefully trim the edges.
- Clean and dry between and under toes. (Never put lotion between toes.)
- Report anything unusual.

Shaving

Shaving is an individual choice. Many men prefer a clean-shaven face. Many women desire to shave their legs and underarms. Check the resident's care plan for any restrictions or precautions regarding shaving.

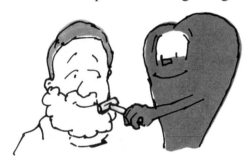

Encourage residents to shave themselves if they are able. If help is needed, shave after bathing when the skin is soft, or use a warm washcloth to soften the skin. Be extremely cautious not to nick the person's skin, and wear gloves to avoid the risk of contact with blood. If you use an electric razor, be sure you know how to use it correctly and safely before you begin.

Follow these guidelines for shaving.

1. Gather all equipment before you begin:
   - razor
   - washcloth
   - towel
   - gloves
   - shaving cream or soap
   - basin with warmwater
2. Wash your hands, and put on gloves.
3. Explain what you are going to do.
4. Help the resident to wash with warm water.

5. Place the towel under the area being shaved, and apply shaving cream.
6. Hold the skin taut, and shave in the direction the hair grows.
7. Gently pat skin dry with the towel.
8. Make the resident comfortable.
9. Clean equipment, and dispose of it properly.
10. Tidy the area.
11. Remove gloves, and wash your hands.

Mouth Care

Poor mouth care leads to cavities, gum disease, mouth infections, and loss of teeth. Mouth problems may affect the resident's ability and desire to eat, resulting in poor nutrition or insufficient fluid intake. Report any redness, white patches, swelling, sores, or bleeding to your supervisor.

Oral hygiene should be done at least twice a day—morning and evening—and after meals if possible. Residents should be encouraged to do this for themselves if possible. When giving oral care always wash your hands and wear gloves.

Following are examples of conditions that need oral care every two hours if the resident is:

- unconscious
- restricted to NPO (nothing-by-mouth) orders
- using a nasogastric tube
- breathing through the mouth
- receiving oxygen by oxygen mask
- feverish

When caring for an unconscious person, the person's head should be elevated and turned to one side. Use lemon glycerin swabs for mouth care. Move the swabs over the tongue, along the gums, over the teeth, inside the cheeks, and on the roof of the mouth. Put lubricant on the lips to prevent drying.

Flossing

Flossing removes plaque (bacteria) that the tooth-brush misses. Teeth should be flossed a minimum of once a day, prior to brushing.

1. Assemble equipment for flossing and brushing:
   - dental floss
   - soft toothbrush
   - cup with water
   - toothpaste
   - emesis basin
   - towel
   - gloves

2. Explain what you are going to do, and provide privacy.

3. Wash your hands, and put on gloves.

4. For mouth care, ensure the resident is sitting upright (45-90 degrees) with a towel across the chest.

5. Break off about 18 inches of floss and wrap most of the length around a finger, wind the rest around the same finger on your other hand.

6. Be gentle, using a sawing motion as you slide the floss between the teeth, towards the base of the tooth. Slip floss slightly under the gumline. Create a "C" shape around the tooth and use up and down sweeping motions on both sides of each tooth.

7. Move to a fresh section of floss, and continue the process until all of the teeth have been flossed.

8. Discard used floss, and proceed with brushing teeth.

Brushing Teeth

Brushing teeth is the most important part of oral hygiene. Good care extends to the gums and tongue.

1. Moisten toothbrush, apply toothpaste, and hold the toothbrush at a 45-degree angle to the gums.

2. Gently clean the entire mouth (tongue, gums, and all surfaces of the teeth).

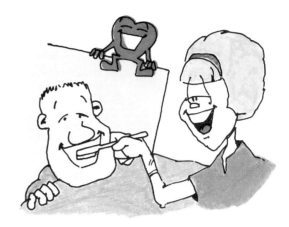

3. Hold an emesis basin at the chin while rinsing the mouth.

4. Dry the person's mouth, and remove the towel.

5. Dispose of supplies properly.

6. Remove gloves, and wash your hands.

7. Report any problems — bleeding, swollen gums, mouth irritations, etc.

Denture Care

Some residents wear full dentures (false teeth) or partials (removable artificial teeth attached to permanent teeth). If a resident complains of discomfort or develops mouth sores, notify your supervisor.

Dentures are easily damaged. After taking the dentures from the resident's mouth, place them directly into a denture cup.

Remove dentures or partials from the mouth for at least eight hours each day. Store them in a clean, labeled denture cup filled with liquid to prevent warping. Be sure to keep them moist whenever they are out of the mouth.

Encourage residents to rinse dentures in cool water after eating and to clean them thoroughly once a day. (Caution: never use hot water, sharp tools, or abrasive toothpaste.) Always handle dentures with care, and assist residents as needed.

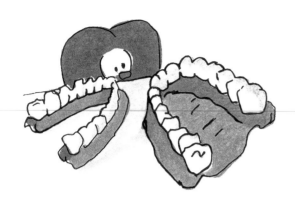

Follow these guidelines for denture care.

1. Assemble supplies before you begin:

    · basin   · denture cup

    · soft denture brush   · denture cleaner

    · soft toothbrush   · drinking glass

    · gloves   · hand towels

2. Wash your hands, and put on gloves.

3. Tell the resident what you are going to do, and provide privacy.

4. Assist the resident with denture removal.

5. Avoid damage to dentures by gently placing them in a denture cup with liquid (e.g., water, cleaning solution). Set cup in a safe location.

6. Place a towel under the resident's chin. Brush and rinse the oral cavity. Pat dry with the towel.

7. Prepare a cleaning area by placing a towel in the sink basin. This will prevent breakage if the dentures are accidentally dropped.

8. Using a soft denture brush, clean all surfaces of the dentures. (Never use a sharp tool or abrasive toothpaste for cleaning.) Rinse well.

9. Gently place dentures in the resident's mouth, or store in the denture cup with fresh, clean liquid.

10. Tidy the area, and store supplies properly.

11. Remove gloves, and wash your hands.

Hair Care

Daily hair care includes brushing and combing. Be sure the comb and brush are clean. Encourage self-care for residents who are able. Assist as needed.

Gently comb or brush tangled hair one section at a time. Place your hand on the person's head to support roots of the hair while brushing or combing. Avoid causing discomfort.

Shampoo hair at least once a week. Check the resident's care plan. If permitted, shampoo during showering. Follow these steps for shampooing hair.

1. Gather all supplies before you begin:

    · mild shampoo   · towel

    · conditioner   · brush

    · wide-toothed comb   · gloves

2. Wash your hands, and put on gloves.

3. Explain what you are going to do.

4. Brush hair gently, removing tangles.

5. Adjust the water temperature for comfort.

6. Wet the hair thoroughly.

7. Shampoo gently, massaging the scalp.

8. Avoid getting shampoo in the eyes and ears.

9. Watch for scalp irritations or problems.

10. Rinse well. Shampoo again if needed.

11. Use conditioner if the resident desires, and rinse thoroughly.

12. Use a wide-tooth comb to ease out tangles; start at the bottom and work toward the scalp.

13. Dry hair immediately. Gently towel dry; then blow dry with warm air.

14. Style in a way the resident desires.

15. Tidy the area, and store supplies properly.

16. Remove gloves, and wash your hands.

17. Report any abnormal observations.

Residents who are confined to their beds may need to be given bed shampoos. There are a variety of devices and supplies to aid with this task. Follow facility guidelines for bed shampoos.

If the facility has a beauty shop, remind residents of their appointments. Help residents to the salon if needed.

Part 2 — Tending to Skin Care

Aging skin needs tender care.

Good skin care is important at any age. It is vital for the elderly. The integumentary (covering) system includes skin, hair, and nails. Skin is the body's largest organ and consists of three layers – epidermis (outer), dermis (middle), and hypodermis (inner – also called subcutaneous).

As skin ages, it becomes thin and fragile, increasing the risk for injury. It loses elasticity, is slower to heal, and provides less insulation. Nerve endings become less sensitive, putting the person at risk of burns, frostbite, etc.

Normal skin is soft, smooth, and pliable. To check elasticity, gently pinch the back of the hand. Skin should resume normal shape when released. If not, hydration needs to be increased. Skin temperature should be the same from head to toe. To check skin temperature, use the back of your hand. Skin color should be uniform.

Abnormal skin conditions include color changes (e.g., paleness, cyanosis, redness, jaundice), sores, rash, scales or dryness, heat, chapping, cracking, blisters, peeling, bruising, and skin tears. Anything abnormal should be reported immediately.

Most elderly people have dry skin. Hydration is very important to prevent cracking, itchiness, and pain. When the skin itches, the person scratches and fragile skin tears easily. Tears allow bacteria to enter the body. Bacteria can cause infection, and fighting infection is especially difficult for the elderly.

Functions of the skin include:

- protecting organs
- providing a barrier to infection
- regulating body temperature
- regulating fluid balance
- producing vitamin D
- storing fat and vitamins
- providing sensation (e.g., heat, cold, pain)
- showing emotions (e.g., blushing when embarrassed, paleness when frightened)

Preventing Skin Problems

NAs help maintain healthy skin by providing gentle care, relieving pressure, controlling moisture, and carefully observing skin for any problems or changes. Use preventive measures by keeping your own nails short and avoid wearing jewelry that could cause injury.

Daily skin care requires vigilant observation. Always check skin for any abnormal conditions including pain, irritation, bruising, or tearing. Careful inspection is required to look for any new sores or growths, and any sores that do not heal. Regularly check feet for corns, calluses, warts, fungal infection, ingrown toenails, blisters, or deformities.

Always check the person's care plan for specific instructions. Anything abnormal should be reported immediately. **Early intervention can prevent serious problems.**

Relieve pressure. Lying or sitting in one position for too long causes pressure that affects the blood supply by reducing circulation to the skin. A resident who is in bed all day needs to change position at least every two hours. A resident in a wheelchair needs to change position every hour or less.

There are many types of pressure reducing devices used to protect the skin over bony areas. These vary from specially designed mattresses to pillows, pads, cushions, and wedges. Bedding must be wrinkle-free, clean, dry, and without particles. Check each resident's care plan for instructions regarding positioning, and follow facility guidelines.

Control moisture. Keep the skin clean and dry. Moisture from urine, feces, and perspiration increases the risk of skin injury. Change underpads frequently, schedule toileting, and expose the resident to air or sunlight if possible. Provide privacy, and always preserve the resident's dignity.

Prevent friction. Avoid rubbing two surfaces together (e.g., skin-to-skin, skin-to-bedding). Lubricate the skin with lotion, and apply powder sparingly where there is skin-to- skin contact. Always be gentle, and never rub the skin vigorously. Avoid sliding or dragging when you move the person in bed.

Prevent shearing (combination of pressure and friction). This usually occurs when a resident is in the Semi-Fowler position and slides toward the bottom of the bed. Shearing bends and closes blood vessels, and lack of adequate blood supply causes tissues to die. Prevent shearing by keeping the head of the bed flat, using sheepskin or heel/elbow protectors, and rolling (not sliding) the resident to remove linen from underneath.

Pressure Points

Continuous pressure of a person's own weight can cause stress to the skin that covers bony areas of the body. These pressure points are at high risk of developing pressure ulcers, which are painful and very difficult to cure. Reduce the risk of pressure ulcers with soft supports and frequent repositioning.

See the illustration below, and check these points carefully to detect early signs of pressure ulcers:

· back of ears	· back of hands
· shoulder blades	· back bone
· elbows	· pelvic bone
· hip bones	· buttocks
· knees	· ankles
· heels	· toes

Pressure ulcers develop in four stages.

- The first sign is skin surface (often over a bony area) that is red, pink, darkened (bruised) or mottled (spots and streaks). The discoloration does not fade within 15 minutes after pressure is released.

- In the second stage, the top layer of skin breaks open. The ulcer may appear as a blister, abrasion, or a shallow basin-like wound.

- In the third stage the skin breaks down. Subcutaneous tissue may be exposed and the sore looks like a deep crater.

- In the fourth stage, the sore penetrates to the muscle or bone, and there is infection and drainage.

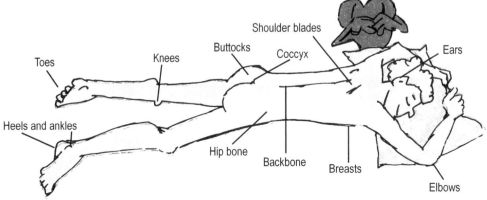

Part 3 — Providing Physical Comfort

Help residents to be as comfortable as possible.

It is important for everyone to meet their personal need for rest. Without enough rest, health problems are likely to develop. Inability to rest may be due to physical, psychological, social, and environmental factors. Observe each resident's physical and mental condition, and report any areas of concern.

Promoting Rest

Provide conditions that are suitable for rest. Use appropriate behavior, movements, and tone of voice to encourage relaxation.

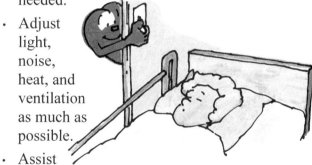

- Talk to the resident and ask what help is needed.
- Adjust light, noise, heat, and ventilation as much as possible.
- Assist the resident into a comfortable position which is consistent with the plan of care.
- Help the resident carry out any required pre-rest routines or activities.
- If monitoring the resident's rest is part of the care plan, keep accurate records.

Seek advice from an appropriate person if you have any difficulties with promoting rest.

Minimizing Discomfort and Pain

Everyone experiences pain or discomfort at times, but the ability to cope is different for each person. Individual beliefs and cultural background often affect the way a person deals with pain or discomfort (e.g., medication, yoga, massage, herbal remedies).

Prevent discomfort or pain as much as possible. Residents should never have to suffer any longer than necessary. Encourage residents in your care to use self-help methods if they are able. Whatever method is used must be in accordance with the care plan.

Follow these guidelines to help minimize pain.

- Encourage residents to express feelings of discomfort or pain, and report any complaints to the nurse.
- If monitoring pain or discomfort is part of the care plan, keep accurate records.
- Position the resident for comfort.
- Explain the methods that are available for controlling discomfort.

Seek advice from an appropriate person if you have any problems dealing with discomfort or pain.

*See Flash Cards for Pain Assessment Tool.

Insomnia

Insomnia is a disorder of initiating and maintaining sleep. Sleep is an important process to remedy "wear and tear" during the waking hours. Before there is any attempt to treat insomnia, a thorough assessment of the causes is essential.

Following are factors that can affect sleep:

- illness, coughing, or pain
- worry or tension
- sleep environment (e.g., comfort, temperature, lighting, noise level)
- hunger or stimulation (e.g., caffeine)
- the need to use the toilet
- interrupted pre-sleep routine

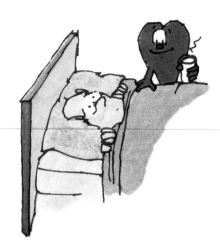

Following are suggestions (if permitted) to promote sleep.

- sleep-compatible bedtime routine (e.g., a hot milky beverage)
- decaffeinated coffee or tea
- not having naps during the day
- relaxation techniques

As a last resort, the doctor may prescribe medication to induce sleep.

Back Rubs

Back rubs help relieve tension and increase circulation. Because aging skin is fragile, back rubs may not be allowed. Follow the policies of the facility where you work.

Always check the care plan before you give a back rub. Restrictions may apply to residents with back injuries, skin problems, and certain heart or lung disorders.

Guidelines for giving back rubs include keeping your fingernails short to prevent scratching and using lotion to prevent friction. Before you begin, warm the lotion in a basin of warm water, and be sure your hands are warm.

Following are steps for giving back rubs.

1. Check the resident's identification, and explain what you are going to do.

2. Wash your hands.

3. Position the resident in a prone or side-lying position that is comfortable and allows good body mechanics.

4. Provide privacy, and expose the resident's back (keeping the rest of the body covered).

5. Observe the back for any skin problems.

6. Apply warmed lotion to the lower back, and use long strokes upward from the waist to the shoulders and over the upper arms; then back across the shoulders, and down the back to the waist using small circular motions.

7. Repeat step 6 for 4-6 minutes.

8. Gently pat the back dry with the towel, and help the resident get dressed.

9. Make the resident comfortable, and place the call signal within easy reach.

10. Tidy the area, and store supplies properly.

11. Wash your hands.

12. Chart the procedure, and report anything abnormal.

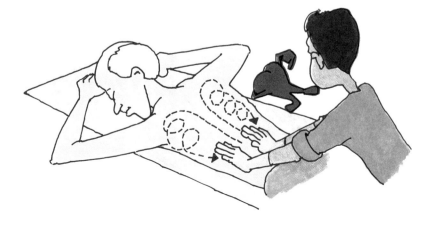

Part 4   Using Bedpans

Provide privacy and minimize the resident's anxiety.

Elimination is the body's natural process for getting rid of waste and is essential for the body to function. The resident who needs help may be embarrassed. It is the NA's job to be professional, provide privacy, and minimize the resident's anxiety.

Assist with toileting as needed, and respond as soon as residents request help. If residents are unable to use the bathroom, provide alternatives.

Bedpans are used for residents who are unable to get out of bed. Women use bedpans for both urination and bowel movements. Men use them for bowel movements only.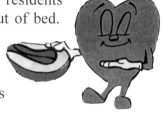

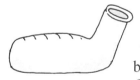 **Urinals** are used by men to urinate. The urinal can be used while lying in bed, standing at bedside, or sitting on the edge of the bed.

Orthopedic (fracture) pans are for residents in traction or casts and for residents who have difficulty moving in bed. Orthopedic pans are shallow on one end and have a thin rim. The shallow end slides under the buttocks with minimum movement.

Following are procedures for using bedpans.

1. Assemble all equipment:

    - gloves
    - hand towel
    - waterproof pad
    - disposable hand wipes
    - warm bedpan and cover
    - wash basin with warm water
    - soap
    - washcloth
    - toilet tissue

2. Wash your hands, and put on gloves.

3. Explain what you are going to do, and provide privacy.

4. Gently place the waterproof pad under the resident.

5. Ask the resident to bend the knees with feet flat on the bed and raise the hips. Assist if needed with your hand under the person's lower back, and place the bedpan.

6. If the resident is unable to raise the hips, roll to side-lying position, place the pan, and roll onto the pan.

7. Help the resident to a sitting position if possible, and cover with a sheet.

8. Place toilet paper and hand wipes within easy reach of the resident.

9. Place the call light within easy reach, and tell the resident to signal when finished.

10. Remove gloves, and raise the head of the bed.

11. Stay nearby to check on the resident, and respond to the call light quickly.

12. When the resident has finished, put on clean gloves.

13. With the bed flat, assist with wiping as needed.

14. Remove the bedpan by turning the resident to the side while holding the pan.

15. Assist with hand washing and positioning.

16. Return to the bathroom, and observe feces for blood or other problems; collect a specimen if needed, and dispose of waste matter in the toilet. Put the lid down and flush.

17. Clean the area, and dispose of equipment in designated areas.

18. Remove gloves, and wash your hands.

19. Chart details, and report any elimination problems or irregularities.

Bedside commodes are for residents who have the ability to get out of bed but cannot use the bathroom. The commode is a chair with a hole in the seat and a bed-pan below. It is used like a toilet, but the pan must be removed and emptied after each use.

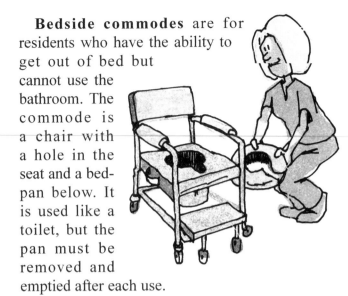

The procedure for using commodes is the same as bedpans with the following exceptions.

- Be sure the bedpan or bucket is placed in the commode.

- If the commode has wheels, be sure wheels are locked.

- Help the resident get out of bed onto the commode, and assist back into bed when finished.

Part 5 Treating Bowel and Bladder Problems

Bladder and bowel problems need special attention.

It is important to observe urine and feces for frequency, amount, color, and odor. Check whether urine is cloudy or clear, and observe the texture of feces. Report any problems or complaints.

Urine is normally pale yellow and clear. Darker yellow usually indicates the need for more fluid. If you notice anything abnormal (e.g., color, odor, blood), report it.

Bowel movements (BM) eliminate bodily waste (feces) through the anus. Frequency of bowel movements varies from person to person and is affected by age, disease, medications, diet, fluids, and activity. The general range is three times a day to three times a week. The NA must document each BM and recognize problems related to elimination. Any abnormal urine or feces should be reported before it is discarded. Report any complaints of pain or burning during elimination.

Constipation is bowel movements that are infrequent and painful with hard feces. Treatment includes adjusting the diet, increasing fluids, and adding physical activity. If these measures are not effective, a suppository or enema may be ordered.

Impaction is a serious form of constipation with inability to pass fecal matter. The resident may complain of pain in the abdomen or rectum. There may be an absence of bowel movements for several days, and small amounts of liquid may be seeping from the anus. Report any symptoms of impaction immediately.

Diarrhea is watery stool. Causes include food irritations, medications, and infections. The urge to eliminate may happen suddenly. Keep a call light/ signal within easy reach of the resident, and respond promptly. Pay extra attention to hygiene, and encourage fluid intake to replace loss of fluids.

Watch for anything unusual and any problems related to elimination. Report any concerns immediately. Elimination problems include the following:

Symptom	Problem
loose feces	diarrhea
dark or "tar" feces	possible internal bleeding
hard feces	constipation
small, infrequent feces	possible impaction
dark or cloudy urine	possible urinary tract infection
pain or burning on urination	possible infection
small, frequent amounts of urine	possible infection

Bowel and Bladder Training

Some residents lose bowel and bladder control. This condition is called **incontinence.** Causes include age, disease, immobility, physical restraints, and confusion. Training programs help residents regain control of elimination. Follow instructions carefully for residents who have training plans. Relearning bowel and bladder control takes time and patience.

The goal of training is to establish regular patterns for elimination and to minimize or eliminate incontinence. Individual schedules are established. In order for training to be successful, instructions must be followed exactly. If training begins in the early stages of incontinence, the resident may improve within six weeks. Others may take a year or more.

All residents need to be offered frequent toileting. Some residents have "accidents" because they are embarrassed to ask for help with elimination needs. Failing to toilet residents who are continent is a form of abuse (forced incontinence). Not providing pericare after residents soil themselves is also abuse. Always be supportive and sensitive to the residents' toileting needs.

Some residents wear special briefs for incontinence. Learn to apply the briefs correctly. Improper use can cause skin problems. Change briefs whenever they are wet or soiled, and clean the skin thoroughly. Discard briefs according to procedures at the facility where you work.

Observe what is happening when incontinence occurs. Sometimes incontinence increases with despair, excitement, anxiety, or isolation; residents are seldom incontinent at social events. Encourage social activities that are useful and interesting, and promote social interaction.

Bladder Retraining

Keep accurate records of fluid intake, and record the time when the resident voids or wets. Provide toileting according to the individual's retraining schedule.

Encourage adequate fluid intake. Unless the care plan states otherwise, provide fluids with meals and between meals. Cutting back on fluid does not decrease incontinence and may cause serious health problems.

Assist with proper positioning. Males void more easily standing, and females void more easily sitting with feet firmly on the floor.

Bowel Retraining

The goal of bowel retraining is to gain control of bowel movements and develop a pattern of elimination. Explain the training program to the resident and encourage cooperation.

Follow each resident's care plan carefully. If allowed, teach exercises that strengthen abdominal muscles. Provide a regular eating schedule, and study eating habits. For residents who are able, encourage ambulation and physical activities.

Find out whether there has been a change in diet, fluid intake, or physical activity. Ask how often and what time of day bowel movements occurred previously.

Explain that every body system depends on water in order to function. Offer water and beverages throughout the day (unless the care plan states otherwise).

Establish a toileting schedule. Bowel evacuation often occurs about a half hour after breakfast. Be sure the resident has easy access to the toilet, or offer bedpans and assistance frequently. Provide privacy, allow sufficient time for toileting, and do whatever is necessary to ensure the resident's comfort and safety.

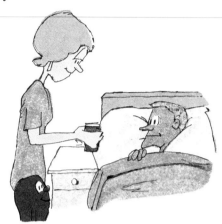

Part 6	**Understanding Digestion**

Aging affects the digestive system.

To understand the elimination process, you need to know how the digestive system processes food. The digestive system is about 30 feet long, extending from the mouth to the rectum.

Digestion begins in the mouth where teeth chew and saliva moistens food for swallowing. Digestion continues in the stomach where acid and digestive enzymes are produced. The small intestine absorbs nutrients from food to nourish the body. Wastes are carried through the large intestine to the rectum. The elimination process rids the body of waste materials through feces and urine.

Following is an overview of the digestive process:

teeth	chew food
salivary glands	lubricate and break down foods
tongue	helps with chewing and swallowing
epiglottis	keeps food out of the lungs
esophagus	moves food to the stomach
liver	aids digestion and stores vitamins
stomach	digests food
gallbladder	stores and releases bile
pancreas	aids digestion and controls insulin
small intestine	absorbs food and water into the bloodstream
large intestine (colon)	reabsorbs water and moves feces along
rectum	holds feces for voluntary elimination
anus	is where feces leave the body

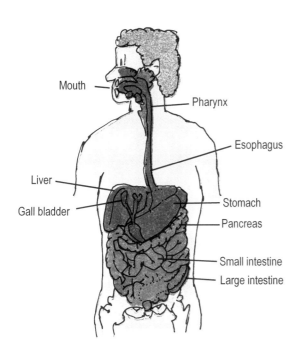

Many people have digestive problems. The digestive system is affected by age, diet, fluids, activity, disease, and medications. As a person ages, food is absorbed more slowly. The ability to taste and smell is reduced and may affect the person's appetite. Some people lose control of their bowels, and others have decreased bowel movements. Report problems related to digestion promptly, including any complaints of abdominal pain or nausea.

Digestive problems include the following:

constipation	infrequent and painful elimination with hard feces
diarrhea	frequent elimination of watery stool
fecal impaction	serious complication of constipation; inability to defecate
anal incontinence	inability to control feces and gas
flatulence	excess gas or air in the stomach or intestines

The **urinary system** plays an important role in removing waste from the bloodstream and producing urine. The system requires sufficient fluids to maintain normal body functioning.

Following is an overview of the urinary system:

kidneys	filter waste from the blood and create urine
ureters	connect the kidneys and the bladder
bladder	stores urine
urethra	passes urine from the bladder, out of the body

Be alert to urinary tract infection (UTI). Symptoms include a burning sensation while voiding, increased frequency, backache, and urine that is cloudy, bloody, or has a strong odor. Report any symptoms promptly.

Summary

Before giving care, always tell the resident what you are going to do. Be familiar with each resident's care plan, and be alert to any restrictions. Offer choices whenever possible, and encourage residents to provide self-care to the extent they are able. Residents have the right to participate in decisions about their care.

Keep residents as comfortable as possible, and ensure their safety at all times. Promote good health, and enhance self-esteem by keeping residents clean and well-groomed. Provide gentle skin care, and reposition residents often. Encourage good oral hygiene. Offer frequent toileting, and be readily available to assist as needed. Avoid embarrassing or offending anyone at any time.

Review

1. Describe three or more safety precautions when assisting residents in bathing.

2. Describe foot care.

3. Explain three or more ways to avoid skin injuries.

4. List five or more pressure points.

5. Explain the use of bedpans, urinals, fracture pans, and bedside commodes.

6. What is impaction, and what are the symptoms?

7. Describe bowel and bladder training programs.

8. How does aging affect the digestive system?

Module 8

Following Care Procedures

Being alert to special needs is vital.

Objectives:

- Explain how to measure intake and output

- Describe specimen collection

- Describe special care for residents with tubing

- Demonstrate proper application of bandages and dressings

- Demonstrate proper bed making

Need-to-Know Words

- intake and output
- edema
- dehydration
- specimen
- enema
- urine
- stool
- sputum
- respiratory
- pulse oximeter
- elimination
- defecate
- catheter
- cyanosis
- flatus
- ostomy
- stoma
- dry dressings
- mitered corners

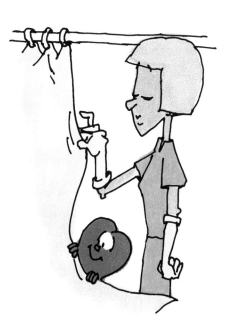

Part 1   Documenting Fluid Intake and Output

Fluid balance is extremely important for good health.

There is no single formula for how much water a person should drink. Needs depend on many factors including health, activity level, body weight, and climate.

Every day the body loses water through breathing, perspiring, urinating, and bowel movements. To function properly, the body needs a daily supply of fluids—water, beverages, and foods that contain water.

Loss of too much water causes dehydration. If the body retains too much water, it causes edema. Both dehydration and edema cause serious health problems.

Dehydration occurs when the body loses more fluid than it takes in. Without enough fluid, the body is unable to carry out normal functions. Warning signs include dark urine, dry "sticky" mouth, lightheadedness, weakness, and increased thirst. Severe fluid loss can become a life-threatening emergency.

The elderly are at risk because they usually do not feel as thirsty as younger people. Keep fresh water at bedside within easy reach, and offer to pour a drink whenever you enter the room (unless the care plan states otherwise). Offer foods such as juices, gelatin, popsicles, ice cream, and broth if the resident's diet allows them. Provide assistance as needed.

Edema (too much fluid in the tissues) may cause painful swelling. Most often it affects the feet, ankles, or legs. It may affect other body parts (e.g., face, hands). Heart and kidney disease, as well as too much salt, can cause edema.

Help residents with edema to be more comfortable by encouraging them to wear loose-fitting clothing. Raising a swollen extremity (limb) above the heart may help relieve pressure and decrease discomfort.

Some residents have special orders from doctors regarding fluids. Sometimes orders are for "restricted fluids;" check the care plan for restrictions. Some orders are to "force fluids;" encourage the resident to drink extra fluids. Orders for "NPO" mean nothing by mouth.

You may be instructed to measure fluid intake and output (I/O) to help monitor a resident's health. It is important to record intake and output as they occur.

Measuring Intake

To get an accurate measurement of intake, it is necessary to record all fluids taken by the resident. Measure fluids taken by mouth and soft foods that turn to liquid at room temperature (e.g., ice cream, gelatin, custard). Intake also includes intraveneous feedings.

- Record intake as soon as it is consumed.
- Record water taken from bedside pitchers.
- Record between-meal beverages (e.g., coffee, tea, juice).

Fluid measurements are usually recorded in cubic centimeters (cc). One ounce equals 30 cc.

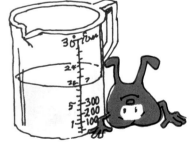

To measure intake, you need to know how much fluid is served. Then measure any leftover fluids, and subtract the amount from what was served. Graduates (containers with marks) are used to measure intake and output. Markings indicate amounts in ounces (oz) and cubic centimeters (cc) or milliliters (mL). Facilities generally provide conversion tables for measurements.

Measuring Output

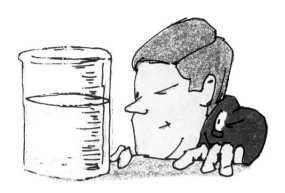

Fluid intake and output should be fairly equal. Output includes urine, watery stool, blood loss, vomitus, wound drainage, and perspiration. Urine is the easiest and most reliable measurement of output.

For an ambulatory resident, a specimen pan is placed on the toilet seat. Tell the resident not to empty the pan. When a resident uses a bedpan, urinal, or commode, the NA removes the sample to the bathroom. Urinary catheter bags are emptied and measured at the end of each shift.

Follow these procedures to measure urine.

1. Assemble all supplies before you begin:
   - gloves
   - I/O record sheet
   - measuring container
   - pen

2. Wash your hands, and put on gloves before handling the bedpan.

3. Pour urine into the measuring container.

4. Put the container on a level surface; at eye-level carefully note the output.

5. Look for anything abnormal in the urine:
   - blood
   - unusual odor or color
   - discharge
   - mucus or sediment

6. Empty the urine into the toilet, put the lid down, and flush.

7. Tidy the area, and dispose of supplies in designated areas.

8. Remove gloves, and wash your hands.

9. Record output, and report any irregularities.

Collecting Specimens

Sometimes blood, body fluid, and waste samples need to be analyzed. You may be asked to collect specimens (samples) of urine, stool, or sputum. Specimens are necessary for observing changes in the resident's physical condition. Use precautions, and follow medical asepsis guidelines. Follow instructions exactly; accuracy is critical.

Before you begin, complete a label with the resident's complete name, date, time, and other requested information. Attach the label to the container.

Stool specimens (feces) are observed for consistency, color, amount, and odor. Record when the specimen was taken and what you observed. Report anything unusual.

Urine specimens provide important information about kidney functions. Instructions for collecting urine may vary:

routine	resident urinates in specimen cup or clean bedpan
midstream clean-catch	clean perineal area; then catch urine midstream (after urination starts and before it stops)
24-hour specimen	save the resident's urine for 24 hours; post notices in the resident's room stating start and finish time; follow facility procedures for storing

Sputum specimens are collected for laboratory tests to check for respiratory (breathing) disorders. Sputum is mucus that is coughed up from the lungs. Early morning is the best time to obtain a sputum specimen.

Part 2 — Dealing with Elimination Problems

Be alert to any changes or difficulties with elimination.

Problems with elimination can be serious. Your observations, records, and reports about elimination are very important. The decisions for treating elimination problems are often based on your records and reports.

Be sure to document all bowel movements. Report any changes in the resident's normal elimination pattern and any complaints of pain or discomfort.

Laxatives and Suppositories

If the resident is unable to defecate (eliminate waste from the bowel), the doctor may order special treatment or medication such as an enema or a laxative. Policies for administering enemas and laxative suppositories vary from facility to facility. Always follow the facility's procedures.

Laxatives are medications that loosen the waste materials in the bowel and make evacuation easier. Laxatives require a doctor's orders. The doctor may order a rectal suppository to stimulate the bowel and lubricate the stool.

Enemas

Enemas are ordered by the doctor to relieve constipation or to clean the bowel prior to special procedures. Regulations vary as to whether NAs give enemas. In some facilities, only licensed nurses or NAs with advanced training provide enemas. Always follow the procedures for the facility where you work.

An enema stimulates the bowel to release waste material by introducing fluid into the rectum. A cleansing enema requires a doctor's order. The solution that is used depends on the reason for the enema. The fluid may be a commercially prepared solution that is ready for use, or you may be instructed to prepare the solution.

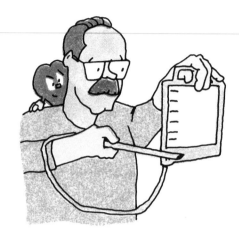

Before you begin any procedure, review the care plan. Be sure you have sufficient training. Always follow instructions very carefully.

1. Assemble all equipment before you begin:
   - bedpan or commode
   - bath thermometer
   - toilet tissue
   - waterproof bed protector
   - enema kit
   - lubricant
   - bath blanket
   - gloves
   - IV pole/stand

2. Wash your hands, and put on gloves.

3. Provide privacy and explain what you are going to do.

4. Prepare the enema as directed.

5. Check the water temperature (generally 105°).

6. Clamp the tubing, and lubricate the tip.

7. Position the enema bag for use (may require an IV pole/stand).

8. Place the waterproof bed protector under the buttocks, and place the bedpan behind the resident.

9. Unclamp the tubing, and allow enough solution to flow into the bedpan to remove air from the tubing.

10. Ask the resident to take a deep breath; as the resident exhales, gently insert the tubing two to four inches into the rectum. Stop if the resident complains of discomfort or you feel resistance. Do not force the tubing.

11. Continue the enema until the amount ordered is given, the resident can no longer tolerate the procedure, or the resident expresses a desire to defecate.

12. Clamp the tubing before the enema bag is empty to prevent air from entering the rectum.

13. Gently withdraw the tubing from the rectum; wrap the tip of the tubing with toilet tissue, and place it inside the enema bag.

14. Help the resident to the bathroom or onto a bedpan or commode, and place the toilet tissue and call signal within easy reach. Ask the resident not to flush the toilet.

15. Leave the room, stay nearby, and answer the call signal promptly.

16. Assist as needed with wiping, perineal care, and hand washing.

17. Make the resident comfortable.

18. Check the elimination for anything abnormal. Then close the toilet lid, and flush.

19. Tidy the area, and dispose of equipment in designated areas.

20. Remove gloves, and wash your hands.

21. Record details.

| Part 3 | **Caring for Residents with Tubing** |

Tubing requires extra caution and care.

Some residents need special tubes to provide liquids, supply oxygen, or eliminate urine. Learn how the tubes work, and be alert to any problems or hazards. Be careful with the tubing whenever you are providing care.

Feeding Tubes

Some residents are fed through tubes because they cannot eat or drink. Tubes are ordered by a doctor.

The tube may be inserted through the nose and into the stomach **(nasogastric tube),** or the tube may go through a small incision directly into the stomach **(gastrostomy tube).** A nutritionally-balanced liquid diet is fed through the tube using a pump.

The NA must be careful when moving, bathing, or dressing a resident with a nasogastric or gastrostomy tube. It is important to provide good care to the area and to prevent pulling on the tube.

A nasogastric tube is securely taped at the nostrils to keep it in place. The connecting tube is fastened at the resident's shoulder to prevent pulling.

Follow these guidelines to care for residents with tubing.

· Watch for any irritation where the tube enters the body.

· Report any signs of discomfort immediately.

· If the tube becomes blocked, report it immediately.

· Keep all foods and beverages away from residents whose care plans indicate NPO (nothing by mouth).

· Always report anything unusual.

Oxygen Tubes

Oxygen or nasal tubes are ordered by the doctor when the resident's body needs more oxygen than it is able to take in by itself. The doctor determines the course of the oxygen therapy and (in most facilities) a licensed nurse administers it. The NA does not make adjustments to a resident's oxygen supply. Instructions may include monitoring oxygen levels with a device called a pulse oximeter (oxygen-measuring device placed on the resident's fingertip or earlobe). Always follow the facility's guidelines.

The nasal cannula has two soft prongs that are inserted into the nostrils approximately one-half inch. A length of tubing connects the oxygen source to the cannula. The NA must be careful that the tubing does not become dislodged at any time.

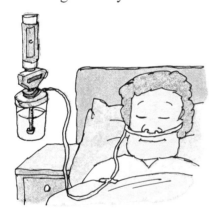

Following are important points for oxygen care.

- Keep the resident's lips, mouth, and nostrils moistened to prevent drying and cracking.

- Be sure the tubing fits comfortably.

- Check tubing frequently to be sure there are no obstructions to oxygen flow.

- Observe the facility's safety rules for oxygen use.

- Immediately report any unusual observations.

Be alert to cyanosis (bluish discoloration) and report it immediately. Cyanosis is a life-threatening condition that indicates low oxygen.

Catheter Tubes

A urinary catheter is a tube inserted through the urethra into the bladder to drain urine from the bladder. An indwelling catheter (also called retention or Foley catheter) remains in the bladder to drain urine continuously into a drainage bag.

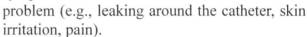

Catheters require a doctor's order and are inserted by licensed staff. An indwelling catheter puts the resident at risk of infection. Special care is necessary to control germs and bacteria. Always be alert to symptoms that could indicate a problem (e.g., leaking around the catheter, skin irritation, pain).

Keep accurate records of intake and output. Notify your supervisor immediately if there is decreased urinary output or if the urine is dark, foul-smelling, or leaves sediment in the catheter tubing, or if there are complaints of tenderness, burning, or pain.

Catheter Care

Always keep the drainage bag below the level of the resident's bladder to prevent urine from going back up the tube. The tubing must be free of kinks and obstructions to allow the urine to flow freely. If the catheter stops flowing, notify your supervisor immediately.

Catheters require daily care. Always check the care plan. Following are basic guidelines.

1. Gather supplies:
   - basin of warm water
   - soap, washcloth
   - hand towel
   - waterproof bed protector
   - bath blanket
   - gloves

2. Check the resident's identification, and explain what you are going to do.

3. Provide privacy, and cover the resident with a bath blanket.

4. Wash your hands, and put on gloves.

5. Place a bed protector under the resident's perineal area.

6. Expose the area around the catheter while keeping the rest of the body covered.

7. Check that the water in the basin is a comfortable temperature, and add soap to a wet washcloth. (Note: some facilities use antiseptic solution packets instead of soap and water.)

8. Gently check and clean the perineal area. Report any sores, redness, leakage, bleeding, or other problems immediately.

9. Hold the catheter near the meatus (opening, passage) to avoid tugging on the catheter. Gently clean and rinse at least four inches of the catheter nearest the meatus. Clean *away* from the area. For each stroke, change to a clean part of the cloth.

10. Holding the catheter near the meatus, gently dry four inches of the catheter, moving away from the meatus.

11. Check that tubing is placed correctly and taped securely.

12. Remove the bed protector and bath blanket, and cover the resident.

13. Make the resident comfortable, and check that the catheter and tubing are not pulling or kinked.

14. Place the call signal within easy reach.

15. Tidy the area, and dispose of linen and supplies in designated areas.

16. Remove gloves, and wash your hands.

17. Record details, and report anything unusual.

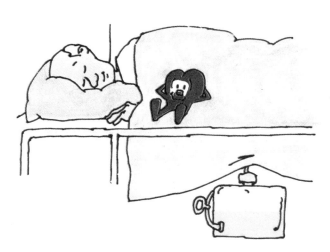

Catheter care may be part of routine morning care, part of pericare, or a separate procedure. Sometimes NAs on each shift perform catheter care. Follow procedures at the facility where you work.

Other Tubes and Appliances

A **rectal tube** is inserted into the rectum to relieve intestinal gas (flatus). A flatus bag is connected to the tube to collect flatus and feces. Your supervisor will tell you if and when someone needs a rectal tube and how long to leave it in place (usually 20 minutes).

An **ostomy** is a surgical procedure that provides an alternate route to eliminate body waste. The opening created by the surgery is called the stoma. Body waste is discharged through the stoma. **Colostomy** and **ileostomy** are two types of ostomies.

After ostomy surgery, residents wear special appliances to collect waste discharged from the stoma. Good skin care is essential to prevent irritation and to keep skin from breaking down around the stoma.

Ostomy patients are taught self-care, and they are encouraged to be as self-managing as possible. Sometimes NAs assist with ostomy care according to individual care plans.

Part 4   Applying Bandages and Dry Dressings

Always wash your hands and use precautions when handling bandages and dressings.

Bandages promote healing and prevent injury. Bandages are applied to extremities to provide comfort, support, and pressure. Commonly used bandages are elastic (also called ace wraps).

Follow these guidelines for proper bandaging.

- Use a bandage of appropriate length and width, and wrap toward the heart (e.g., wrist to elbow, toes to knee) with firm (not tight) and even pressure, keeping the extremity in proper alignment, with good circulation.
- Expose fingers and toes if possible to check circulation.
- Report the time the bandage was applied, the area that was bandaged, and any unusual observations.
- Check the extremity often for color, pain, temperature, swelling, or numbness; report any problems immediately.
- Reapply the bandage if it loosens, moves, or wrinkles.

Dressings are materials used to cover wounds. They protect the wounds and prevent germs from infecting wounded areas. Nursing Assistants provide care for closed wounds by applying clean, dry dressings. Licensed staff generally provide care for open wounds.

Follow these guidelines for applying a dressing.

- Clean and dry the affected area before applying the dressing.
- Avoid touching the part of the dressing that covers the wound.
- Tape the ends of the dressing with tape that can be easily removed without damaging fragile skin.
- Report any unusual observations such as sores, broken skin, discoloration, or bruises.
- Apply lotions (e.g., moisturizers) only to skin that is intact.
- Follow facility procedures for safe disposal of dressings.

Part 5   Making Beds

A properly made bed adds to the resident's comfort and well-being.

Before removing bedding, always check for any belongings (e.g., dentures, clothing). Keep soiled linen away from you, and use linen-handling precautions to prevent contamination. Following are procedures for making an **unoccupied bed.**

1. Gather equipment, and put it on a chair near the bed in the order you will use it:

   - plastic laundry bag
   - pillowcase
   - mattress pad
   - blanket
   - 2 sheets
   - bedspread
   - drawsheet (if needed)

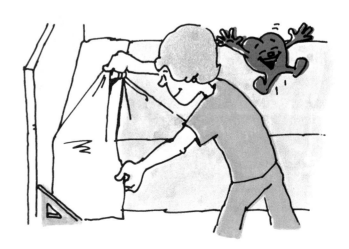

2. Remove used linen, and dispose of it properly.

3. Unfold and lay the bottom sheet so it hangs evenly on both sides.

4. Tuck top of the sheet under the mattress.

5. Make a mitered corner:

   - Pick up the hanging side of the sheet edge about 12 inches from the end of the mattress. Lay it back on the mattress in a triangle fold.

   - Tuck the hanging corner of the sheet under the mattress.

   - Bring the triangle down, and tuck it under the mattress.

6. When the bottom sheet is wrinkle-free, place the top sheet, and miter the corners at the foot. Do not tuck the bottom under the mattress.

7. Make a toe pleat (two- to four-inch fold across the foot area to make room for toes).

8. Place the blanket, then the bedspread, and tuck in the top sheet, blanket, and bedspread together, making mitered corners.

9. Move to the opposite side and repeat, pulling linen tightly to remove wrinkles.

10. Open the pillowcase. Guide the pillow in with seam end first. (Do not hold the pillow under your chin!)

11. Fold extra material under the pillow, and place the pillow on the bed.

12. Place the call signal within easy reach.

Making an **occupied bed** is much the same as making an unoccupied bed with the following exceptions.

1. Get help if needed.

2. Explain to the resident what you are going to do, and provide privacy.

3. Loosen the bed linen, leaving the top sheet to cover the resident.

4. With the far side rail up and locked*, gently roll the resident away from you toward the far side.

5. Roll the used linen toward the resident, and tuck the linen under his or her back.

6. Unfold and place clean linen with the center crease in the center of the bed, and tuck in with mitered corners.

7. Raise the side rail* where you have been working, and move to the opposite side.

8. Lower the rail where you are working, and move the resident onto the clean linen.

9. Remove soiled linen and repeat the process, pulling linen tight and wrinkle-free.

10. Place the clean top sheet over the resident, and pull the soiled sheet from below, keeping the resident covered.

11. Make a toe pleat, replace the blanket and bedspread, and change the pillowcase.

12. Position the resident, put the side rail down, and place the call signal within easy reach.

13. Dispose of used linen properly.

*Beds are equipped with side rails that can be raised to keep residents safe. However, a raised side rail is classified as a restraint. Always follow facility procedures for using side rails.

Summary

NA care procedures include everything from maintaining fluid balance to making beds correctly. Decisions for treating elimination problems are often based on the NA's observations and records. Extra care, caution, and cleanliness are required for residents with special tubing. NAs apply bandages and dry dressings to promote healing and prevent infection.

Review

1. What are the signs of edema?

2. What is dehydration, and how can it be prevented?

3. Describe procedures for measuring intake.

4. Describe procedures for measuring output.

5. Identify five or more important points regarding care of tubes.

6. Explain guidelines for bandaging.

7. Explain guidelines for applying a dressing.

8. Explain safety precautions for making an occupied bed.

Module 9

Taking Vital Signs

Accurate measurements help determine a person's physical condition.

Objectives:

- Name the vital signs
- Identify four locations for measuring temperature
- Explain how to use thermometers
- Identify pulse points
- Demonstrate how to count respirations
- Demonstrate how to take blood pressure

Need-to-Know Words:
- vital signs
- pain assessment
- temperature
- aural
- tympanic
- pulse
- radial
- carotid
- apical
- stethoscope
- respiration
- blood pressure
- sphygmomanometer
- systolic
- diastolic
- hypertension
- hypotension

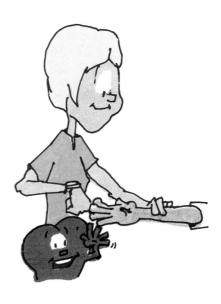

Part 1   Understanding Vital Signs

Vital signs provide valuable information for care and treatment.

Vital signs are measurements of basic body functions to give an indication of health status. The standard vital signs are as follows:

- temperature
- pulse
- respiration
- blood pressure

The medical abbreviations used are VS (vital signs), TPR (temperature, pulse, respiration), and BP (blood pressure). Vitals may also be noted as TPR/BP.

Sometimes the medical community refers to pain as the fifth vital sign. Since pain is not visible, it is difficult to measure. Attention should be given to pain as rated by the person on a scale of 0 (no pain) to 10 (extreme pain). It is important to locate pain and document findings so that it can be treated promptly.
*See Flash Cards for Pain Assessment Tool.

Accurate measurements provide important information that is useful in detecting and monitoring medical problems. Changes in vital signs indicate changes in the person's physical condition. Report any changes immediately. Always check the resident's care plan for any restrictions. An example might be, "Take BP on left arm only, due to mastectomy on right side." Follow facility guidelines and record vital signs accurately.

Part 2   Taking a Temperature

Body heat provides important health information.

Measuring body temperature is one of the basic steps of tracking a resident's vital signs. A temperature higher than normal could be a sign of illness, infection, or other health conditions. An abnormally low temperature may indicate serious health issues. The information also indicates whether a medication or treatment is working (e.g., antibiotic).

Body temperatures vary from person to person. An oral temperature of 98.6°F (37.0°C) is considered the average normal. A person's temperature can vary a degree and still be within normal range. Body temperature can change slightly depending on many factors (e.g., physical activity, time of day, strong emotion, medications, air temperature, and humidity). An elderly person is likely to have a lower-than-average temperature due to the aging process and decreased physical activity. Following are common ways to measure body temperature including average readings and range.

Body area	Average °F	Range°
oral (mouth	98.6°	97.0°–99.0°
rectal (anus)	99.6°	98.6°–100.0°
tympanic (ear)	99.6°	98.6°–100.0°
axillary (armpit)	97.6°	96.6°–98.0°

Both Fahrenheit and Celsius scales are used to measure temperature in medical facilities located within the United States. Measurement in degrees Celsius is the standard in most other countries. Abbreviations relating to temperature are (°) degrees, (F) Fahrenheit, and (C) Celsius.

*See Flash Cards for Temperature Conversion Chart.

Before measuring body temperature, wait at least one hour after exercise or a hot bath. Allow at least 20 minutes after eating, drinking hot or cold liquid, or smoking. The resident should sit or lie in a comfortable position to minimize effects of stress on the reading. If the temperature reading is abnormal or changes from a resident's "normal" measurement, report it immediately.

Thermometers

Thermometers come in a variety of different styles. Learn correct use, placement, cleaning, and storage of the type of thermometers that are used in the facility where you work.

Digital thermometers are simple to use, give quick results, and measurements are in easy-to-read numbers. In the past, mercury-filled glass thermometers were common. They are no longer recommended due to the toxic risk of mercury if the glass breaks.

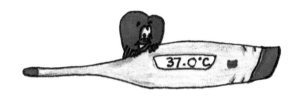

All thermometers require preparation and cleanup procedures. Before you begin, always check the care plan for any restrictions for temperature measurement. Assemble supplies. Tell the resident what you are going to do, and assist to a comfortable position. Then wash your hands, and put on gloves. After measuring temperature, remove and read the display. Clean the thermometer, and place it in the designated area. Dispose of the gloves, and wash your hands. Record the temperature in the resident's chart and report any abnormal readings.

Oral Temperature

An oral temperature may only be taken when a person is able to hold the thermometer securely under the tongue. To get an accurate reading, the person must be able to breathe through the nose.

Never take an oral temperature when a person:

- is unconscious
- has seizures
- is on oxygen
- is less than five years old
- is confused
- is disoriented
- is overcome by coughing or vomiting
- cannot breathe with the mouth closed

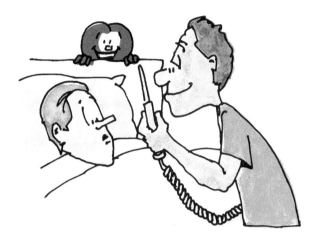

Guidelines for taking an oral temperature:

1. Hold the thermometer at the stem and clean probe end with an alcohol swab.

2. Place a disposable cover over the probe end.

3. Turn device on.

4. Gently insert the probe under the tongue, and ask the resident to keep the lips closed tightly (without biting down).

5. Leave the thermometer in place until the beep, usually about one minute.

6. Eject the disposable cover into the trash.

Rectal Temperature

When you cannot take an oral temperature, you may be directed to take a rectal temperature. Check the care plan for any restrictions. Thermometers used rectally are designated "Rectal Use Only." Always wear gloves, practice medical asepsis, and provide privacy. Support the resident, and prevent any movement that could cause injury.

Guidelines for taking a rectal temperature:

- Place the resident in a side-lying position with the top knee flexed (bent).
- Apply lubricant to the probe end of the thermometer.
- Gently insert the tip about one inch into the rectum; do not force.
- Hold in place until the beep, about one minute.
- Remove and wipe with a tissue.

Tympanic Temperature

The tympanic thermometer uses infrared technology to measure temperature inside the ear canal. It reads the heat of the tympanic membrane (eardrum). This method gives a fast reading, and it is simple and less invasive to use.

Guidelines for taking an aural (ear) temperature:

- Use a new ear probe jacket each time, and follow the operating instructions carefully.
- Gently tug on the ear, pulling it back. This will help straighten the ear canal, and make a clear path to the eardrum (tympanic membrane).
- Gently insert the thermometer until the ear canal is fully sealed off.
- Press and hold down the button for one second.

Axillary Temperature

Body temperature can be measured at the armpit when you cannot take an oral or rectal temperature (axillary measurement is less accurate).

Guidelines for taking an axillary temperature:

- Place the thermometer in the center of the axilla (armpit).
- Place the resident's arm snugly against the body to hold the thermometer in place.
- Leave the thermometer in place until the beep, about 1 minute.

Other Thermometers

There are other methods for measuring temperature. Using infrared technology, no-touch forehead thermometers read the skin without the need for contact. Temporal scanners measure the heat of the skin surface over the temporal artery on the forehead. Forehead strips are disposable plastic thermometers that change color based on body temperature. The following information regarding glass thermometers is provided if there is no other method available.

Glass Thermometers

The thin glass tube has an inner red or blue line that indicates temperature. Each long mark on the thermometer indicates one degree. Short marks equal two-tenths of a degree.

Use the same procedure as a digital thermometer except for the following:

- Always inspect a glass thermometer for chips or cracks.
- Hold the thermometer firmly by the stem, and shake it down to 96°F or lower.
- Leave the glass thermometer in place for five minutes. Do not leave the resident unattended.
- Remove the thermometer, and hold it at eye level to read the number where the colored line ends in the display window.

Abnormal Temperatures

Elevated temperature may be caused by:	**Subnormal** temperature may be caused by:
· infection	· excessive bleeding
· pain, emotions	· shock
· dehydration	· burns
· warm surroundings	· cold surroundings
· drinking hot fluids	· drinking cold fluids

Follow facility procedures for charting temperatures. Report any significant changes from previous readings.

Part 3   Measuring the Pulse

Pulse rate, rhythm, and force provide vital information.

The heart's contractions (pulse) are measured to determine how fast the heart is beating. The average range for adults is 60-100 beats per minute (bpm).

An irregular pulse may indicate health problems. Measuring the pulse, requires three observations:

- **rate** (number of beats per minute)
- **rhythm** (how regular and even the beats are)
- **strength/force** (weak or pounding)

The pulse can be felt easily at the points of the body where the arteries are closest to the skin. The three most common points are radial, carotid, and apical. Measure the pulse when the resident is resting.

Following are steps for measuring the pulse.

1. Tell the resident what you are going to do.

2. Locate the pulse.

3. Using a watch that displays seconds, count the beats for one full minute. If the beat is irregular, take another reading.

4. Record accurate pulse count. (If you are unsure, measure again.)

5. Report readings that are abnormally low or high and any major changes from previous readings.

Increased pulse rate may be caused by:

- exercise
- heat application
- pain
- heart condition
- fever
- illness
- emotions
- caffeine

Decreased pulse rate may be due to:

- rest
- certain illnesses
- medications

The **radial** pulse is felt in the wrist (on the thumb side). Gently place two fingers over this artery, while supporting the person's forearm.

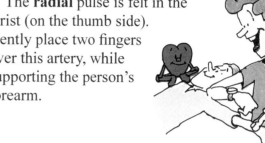

The **carotid** artery is in the neck (in the groove next to the Adam's apple). This method is used for CPR or when the pulse is too weak to feel at the wrist. Pressure on the carotid artery can interfere with the heart's rate and rhythm.

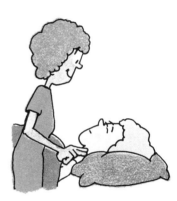

The **apical** pulse is a measurement of heartbeats at the apex of the heart, under the left breast. A stethoscope is needed to hear the apical pulse.

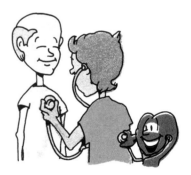

Following are additional sites for measuring pulse:

- temporal (temples)
- popliteal (knee)
- brachial (inside elbow)
- pedal (top of foot)
- femoral (groin)

Part 4 — Counting Respirations

Changes in breathing may be warning signs of respiratory problems.

Respiration is breathing air into and out of the lungs. Each respiration (breath) has two parts:

- inspiration (breathing in)
- expiration (breathing out)

One inspiration and one expiration equal one respiration. To count respirations, watch or feel the resident's chest rise and fall for one full minute. Count respirations when the resident is resting. The average respiratory rate for adults is 14-20 per minute.

Try to observe respirations without the resident's awareness. Do not tell the person that you are counting respirations because it may cause the person to breathe at a different rate than normal. You might pretend to be taking a pulse while you are actually counting respirations. Observe the resident for any breathing problems.

Count respirations for a full minute. Notify your supervisor immediately if there are any irregularities in breathing. Breathing problems may indicate an emergency. Pay special attention to signs of respiratory problems:

- very fast or very slow
- noisy (describe the sound)
- shallow (very little chest movement)
- shortness of breath
- labored (wheezing or with great effort)
- blue color (cyanosis) around lips, nose, or fingernails

Increased respiration may be caused by fever, emotions, exercise, or infections. Decreased respiration may be due to medications or illness.

Part 5 — Measuring Blood Pressure

The heart pumps blood, creating pressure against the arterial walls.

Blood pressure (BP) varies from person to person, and it can change from minute to minute. Age, heredity, and physical condition affect blood pressure. Exercise and stress also affect blood pressure. Blood pressure readings provide valuable information for the care and treatment of the resident.

BP is measured with a sphygmomanometer (blood pressure cuff) and a stethoscope. Cuffs come in various sizes, ranging from child size to large adult. The sphygmomanometer gauge measures blood pressure in mmHg (millimeters of mercury). Each short line represents 2 mmHg, and each long line represents 10 mmHg.

Blood pressure measures at two points—systolic and diastolic pressure. To record blood pressure, systolic is written before diastolic (e.g., 120/80).

Systolic pressure is maximum pressure when the heart contracts and pumps blood. Systolic pressure is higher and is heard first. Normal range for adults is 120 mmHg or less.

Diastolic pressure is minimum pressure when the heart relaxes and pressure decreases. Normal range for adults is 80 mmHg or less.

Allow 15 minutes or more for the resident to rest before measuring blood pressure. Never put a cuff on an arm with an injury or an IV. Always check the individual care plan.

Follow these steps for measuring blood pressure.

1. Gather all equipment before you begin:
   - sphygmomanometer (with correct size cuff)
   - stethoscope
   - antiseptic wipes
   - pen and paper

2. Position the resident comfortably—sitting or lying down—with the resident's arm resting level with the heart. Allow a few minutes of quiet relaxation before measuring BP.

3. Use antiseptic wipes to clean the earpieces and diaphragm of the stethoscope.

4. Supporting the person's arm, straighten it with the palm up. With your fingers, locate the brachial pulse (inside of bent elbow).

5. Wrap the BP cuff snugly around the resident's bare arm, with the cuff's bottom edge one inch above the bend in the elbow; center the positioning mark over the brachial artery.

6. Put the stethoscope eartips in your ears. Place the chestpiece (bell) over the brachial artery.

7. Close the valve. Squeeze the bulb to inflate the cuff past the point that you no longer hear the pulse (about 160 mmHg). Note the number. (If you still hear the pulse, inflate the cuff an extra 30mm—no higher than 200 mmHg).

8. Listen carefully as you open the valve, and let air escape slowly until you hear the first pulse sound. Note the gauge reading for systolic pressure.

9. Continue to let the air out slowly and evenly until the pulse sound disappears. Note the gauge reading for diastolic pressure.

10. Rapidly deflate the cuff, and remove it. If you miss a reading, or need to take another reading, completely remove the cuff. Have the resident raise the arm and flex the fingers. Wait one minute for normal circulation to resume.

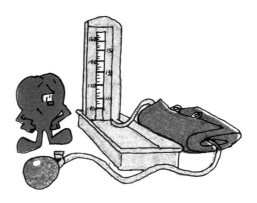

11. Promptly record the systolic and diastolic readings. (Avoid any comments about results that might alarm the resident.)

12. Clean and store equipment properly, and wash your hands.

13. Report anything abnormal or any major change from previous readings.

Hypertension is abnormally high blood pressure (HBP). The higher the pressure, the greater the risk of stroke or heart attack. Elderly people tend to have higher blood pressure due to thickening and hardening of the arteries (arteriosclerosis).

Hypotension is abnormally low pressure. Some people with low blood pressure experience complications (e.g., dizziness, fainting).

Blood Pressure	Systolic	Diastolic
Normal	Below 120	Below 80
High normal	120-139	81-89
Stage 1 HBP	140-159	90-99
Stage 2 HBP	160 or higher	100 or higher

Summary

Vital signs—temperature, pulse, respiration, and blood pressure—provide important information about each resident's physical condition. Accurate measurements are important for determining treatment and evaluating care. Learn to recognize changes, including pain, that indicate problems. Report abnormal measurements and significant changes immediately.

Review

1. Identify four areas to measure body temperature.

2. What is the normal temperature range for adults?

3. Identify three or more circumstances when you would not take an oral temperature.

4. List three observations when taking a pulse.

5. Identify three common areas for measuring pulse.

6. What could cause increased respirations?

7. List four or more breathing irregularities, and explain what you would do.

8. What is hypertension?

Module 10

Following Safety and Emergency Procedures

Simple precautions prevent serious injuries.

Objectives:

- Discuss accident prevention
- Define first aid
- List life-threatening emergencies
- Discuss the purpose of CPR
- Demonstrate abdominal thrusts
- Discuss the use of protective devices
- Describe alternatives to restraints

Need-to-Know Words:

- catastrophe
- first aid
- life-threatening
- shock
- cardiopulmonary resuscitation
- rescue breathing
- airway
- obstruction
- abdominal thrusts
- protective devices
- restraints

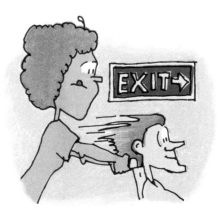

Part 1	Preventing Accidents

The best way to avoid an accident is to be alert to all safety hazards.

Be alert to safety hazards, and take extra precautions to protect elderly and frail people from injury. Following are physical conditions related to aging and illness that put people at risk of accidents:

- poor eyesight
- poor hearing
- osteoporosis (loss of calcium from bones; bones can break very easily, sometimes even without trauma)
- decreased muscle strength
- decreased blood pressure when changing position (orthostatic hypotension)
- irregular heartbeat (causing dizziness, loss of balance)
- paralysis
- dementia
- reduced sense of smell and touch
- side effects of medications (e.g., loss of balance, drowsiness, confusion)

Being Alert to Hazards

Safety awareness can prevent serious injuries. Be alert to the types of accidents that can occur. If something seems wrong, report it. It is better to be wrong than to wait until the problem is out of control.

Preventing Falls

Falls are the leading cause of injury for the elderly. You can help prevent falls and bruises.
- Wipe up spills immediately.
- Keep the call signal close to the resident, and respond to the signal promptly.
- Use proper lighting.

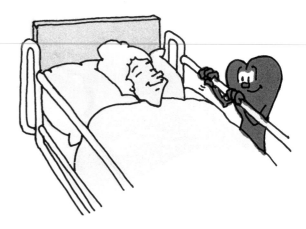

- Use side rails as necessary (if allowed).
- Keep items that are used frequently close at hand so the resident won't fall reaching for them.
- Remove obstacles to walking (e.g., personal items, cords, equipment).
- Assist residents into and out of the bath if needed; never leave them unattended.
- Lock wheels when transferring residents (e.g., wheelchairs, beds).
- Promote ambulation to maintain strength, and assist as needed.
- Encourage use of non-slip footwear.
- Be alert to furniture or objects that pose safety hazards.
- When moving a wheelchair, do not let the resident's feet drag on the floor; use footrests.
- Watch for signs of weakness or dizziness.
- Ensure correct use of assistive devices (e.g., crutches, walkers, canes).
- Encourage residents to use handrails when walking.

Preventing Accidental Poisoning

Accidental poisoning can be the result of carelessness, confusion, or not being able to read labels because of poor vision. Keep all cleansing products and disinfectants locked in storage cupboards.

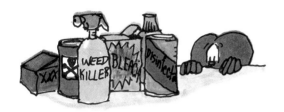

Preventing Burns

Leading causes of burns are cigarettes, bath water, and hot liquids. Following are guidelines to prevent burns.

- Prevent cigarette burns by enforcing smoking restrictions.
- Assist residents with hot foods and liquids.
- Make sure bath water is not too hot. Test the water, and then ask the resident to test the water.

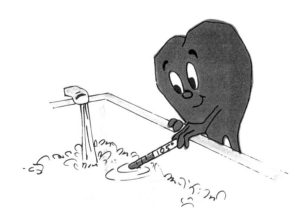

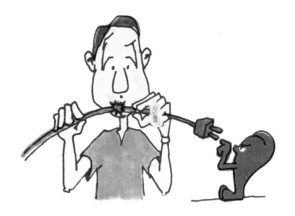

Preventing Electrical Shock

Follow these guidelines to prevent electrical shock.

- Inspect electrical items for damage (such as frayed cords).
- Operate equipment according to instructions. If in doubt, ask.
- Always use properly grounded equipment.
- Be sure people and areas are dry before plugging in equipment.
- Do not overload circuits.
- Do not use extension cords.

Preventing Choking

Some residents are at risk of choking. Be alert to the possibility of choking, especially when residents are eating. Follow these guidelines to avoid choking.

- Supervise residents at meal times.
- Position residents upright (45-90 degrees) for eating.
- Make sure dentures are in if needed.
- Cut food into bite-sized pieces.
- Encourage residents to eat slowly and take small bites.

Be prepared to perform the abdominal thrust procedure if necessary. (See page 95.)

Part 2	Promoting Fire Safety

Be sure you know fire emergency procedures before disaster strikes.

All care facilities have disaster plans. Be prepared before disaster strikes by understanding emergency procedures and participating in fire drills at the facility where you work. Fire prevention is everyone's job.

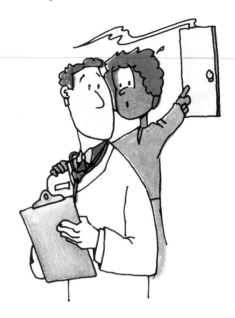

> **In Case of Emergency**
> Stay calm and take immediate action
> to remove residents from danger.

Fire Hazards

Awareness of fire hazards is the first step in prevention. By removing any of these elements, a fire can be prevented:

heat: flame or spark

oxygen: normal air

fuel: any combustible material (items that catch fire and burn easily)

Alert your supervisor immediately if you smell smoke or if a door feels hot. **Do not open the door!**

Smoking

Never leave smokers unattended. Some residents may not be able to handle smoking materials safely. Smoking materials should be stored for safekeeping. Follow the facility's smoking restrictions.

- Restrict smoking to authorized areas only.
- Use noncombustible ashtrays.
- Be sure contents are cool when emptying ashtrays.
- Never use paper cups or garbage bins for ashtrays.
- **Never permit smoking where oxygen is in use.**

Storage

Storage areas are fire hazards. Never store oily rags, paint cans, chemicals, or other combustibles in closed areas.

Aerosol Cans

Never burn aerosol cans, the container might explode. Never use an aerosol spray near open flames or cigarettes, the spray could ignite.

Faulty Wiring

Faulty wiring and equipment are hazards. Inspect all equipment that you use, and report any defects. Do not use frayed power cords, overloaded circuits, overheated equipment, or equipment that is improperly grounded.

In Case of Fire

In case of fire, stay calm. Fire can be a panic situation, and the residents depend on you for their safety. Be sure you know fire and evacuation procedures before disaster hits.

- Know the location of all exits and stairways
- Know the location of fire alarms and extinguishers, and know how to use them.
- Know emergency telephone numbers.

Stop, drop, and roll are important procedures to remember. If clothing catches on fire, stop immediately, drop to the ground, and roll to smother the flames.

Different types of **fire extinguishers** are used for different types of fires. For electrical fires, use a multipurpose extinguisher. Oil and grease fires require a dry chemical. Use water to extinguish paper and wood fires. Never use water on electrical, oil, or grease fires. Using the wrong type of extinguisher for the wrong type of fire can be life-threatening.

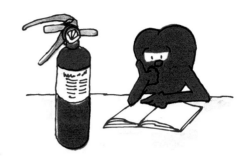

To remember how to use a fire extinguisher:
P-A-S-S
Pull - Aim - Squeeze - Sweep

In case of fire, remember: *RACE!*

R–Rescue
A–Alarm
C–Contain
E–Extinguish

R   A   C   E

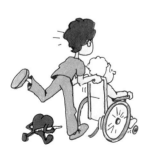

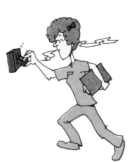

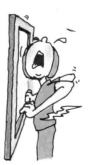

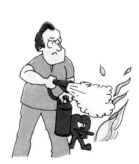

Rescue any residents in immediate danger.

Sound the **Alarm.**

Contain the fire by closing doors and windows.

Extinguish the fire if it is small and you are safe. (Otherwise, let the fire department extinguish it.)

Part 3 — Managing Catastrophes

Take appropriate action whenever safety and security are at risk.

A catastrophe is a sudden disaster that causes a great amount of damage, loss, or destruction. In addition to fires, examples of disasters are earthquakes, hurricanes, floods, and explosions. If a catastrophe strikes, you must be prepared to act quickly, safely, and calmly. Action depends upon the nature of the catastrophe and the facility's disaster plan.

Emergency Procedures

The best defense against a catastrophe is being prepared. Know the facility's emergency procedures BEFORE an emergency strikes.

- Understand rescue and evacuation procedures for the facility where you work.
- Know the location of all exits and stairways.
- Know where fire alarms and extinguishers are located.
- Follow your supervisor's instructions.

After the residents are secured, the NA should report to the supervisor for further instructions. Be prepared to act calmly and professionally under the direction of your supervisor. Take appropriate action immediately.

Instructions might include the following.
- Alert the fire department, police, or Red Cross.
- Evacuate the facility.
- Assist and observe residents.
- Move supplies, equipment, and medical records to a safe place.
- Help with emergency record-keeping.

Earthquakes and Other Catastrophes

In case of an earthquake, stay calm and use common sense. One of the biggest hazards of an earthquake is broken glass. Stay away from windows. Take shelter under a table or in a corner away from windows, mirrors, chimneys, and heavy objects.

After the shaking stops, rescue the residents as directed. Rescue procedures will depend upon the extent of damage caused by the earthquake.

Any unusual occurrences must be reported to the local district office of the Department of Health Services. Be familiar with local emergency numbers, and follow the facility's reporting procedures.

Advance warning is usually available for hurricanes, tornados, and floods. Follow the emergency procedures for the facility where you work. Take appropriate action to provide safety and security.

In Case of Earthquake

DROP to the ground (before the **earthquake** drops you!). **TAKE COVER** by getting under a sturdy desk or table, and **HOLD ON** to it until the shaking stops.

courtesy of www.ready.gov

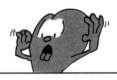

In case of earthquake, remember:

- **DROP**
- **TAKE COVER**
- **HOLD ON**

Part 4 — Responding to Emergencies

Save lives by responding quickly.

Top priority in any emergency is to protect yourself and the residents from immediate danger. The first step is to assess the situation. Consider whether it is safe for you to enter the area. The second step is to assess any victims. Find out whether the person is unconscious or just sleeping by tapping the person and asking loudly, "Are you okay?" If there is no response, assume the person is unconscious and you have an emergency situation.

Good first-aid skills can mean the difference between life and death. Someone's life may depend on you, and you must act fast.

Principles of First Aid

First aid is emergency care for a person who is sick or injured until medical help arrives. First aid is given to prevent death or to keep injuries from getting worse. Get help as soon as possible. Continue first-aid procedures until help arrives.

In any emergency situation, keep the person lying down. Check that there is no immediate danger to you or the victim. Do not move the person except to get away from danger. Offer help and comfort, and keep the person calm and quiet.

Act quickly, giving priority to the most urgent conditions. Tend to life-threatening emergencies in priority order:

1. breathing
2. cardiac arrest
3. severe bleeding
4. severe head injuries
5. open wounds at the chest or abdomen
6. severe shock

Recovery Position

The recovery position may be necessary to prevent choking (aspirating vomitus) or to promote breathing (preventing a collapsed airway), especially if the person is unconscious and lying on his or her back. If you suspect spinal injury, the risk of causing permanent injuries must be considered. Moving is NOT advised unless absolutely necessary.

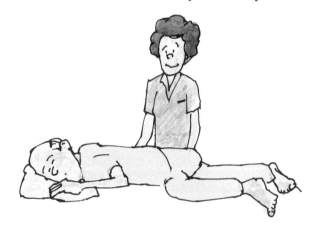

1. Kneel beside the victim and place both of the person's arms close to his or her body.

2. Turn the person gently onto the side.

3. Draw the upper arm and leg upwards and outwards to form right angles with the body. This prevents the person from rolling forward.

4. Pull the underneath arm out gently behind the person. This prevents the person from rolling backward.

Shock

All casualties experience a certain amount of shock. It is important for you to recognize the signs and symptoms of shock. A person in shock may have some or all of the following symptoms.

- The person feels sick, vomits, or may be thirsty.

- The skin is pale, cold, clammy, and may be sweating.

- Breathing becomes shallow and rapid, with yawning and sighing.

- Pulse rate becomes quicker, but weaker.

- Unconsciousness may develop.

Treatment for Shock

Treatment is aimed at getting an adequate supply of blood to the vital organs. Follow these guidelines to treat a person in shock.

- Reassure the person.

- Lay the person down, and raise the legs if possible.

- Place in the recovery position if the person becomes unconscious.

- Keep the person warm.

- Loosen tight clothing to help circulation and breathing.

- Moisten the lips if the person is thirsty (but do not give anything to drink).

- Avoid moving the person unnecessarily.

- Begin cardiopulmonary resuscitation if breathing or heartbeat stops.

Cardiopulmonary Resuscitation

The following is an overview of the purpose and value of cardiopulmonary resuscitation (CPR). **This basic information is NOT A CPR COURSE.** If you are not currently CPR certified (Health Care Provider level) ask the instructor about CPR/AED classes in your area, or check with appropriate training organizations (e.g., American Heart Association, American Red Cross). Procedures change, and it is important to be current.

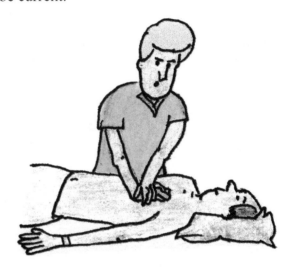

CPR is a valuable life-saving skill. It is an emergency procedure combining chest compressions and rescue breathing when the heart and/or lungs have stopped working. CPR manually keeps oxygenated blood flowing to the brain and other vital organs until normal heart rhythm can be restored.

When performing CPR, think of yourself as a mechanical heart pump for the person. If compressions pause or stop, so does blood flow. Prompt response, quality CPR, and the proper use of an AED may save a life!

It is important that you understand the policies and procedures to activate the Emergency Medical System (EMS) in the facility where you work. There may be other considerations before beginning CPR such as Do Not Resuscitate (DNR) for residents with valid orders.

Survival rate falls rapidly when the start of CPR is delayed. Immediately begin CPR on a person who is unresponsive and not breathing or has abnormal breathing (e.g., gasping and/or extremely labored respirations). It is likely the heart has stopped pumping (cardiac arrest). Every second counts; brain damage occurs within four to six minutes, and death may occur within ten minutes when deprived of oxygen.

The American Heart Association (AHA) changed guidelines in 2010 emphasizing quality chest compressions ahead of airway and breathing (referred to as the C-A-B for CPR). Following are the order, actions, and general guidelines for CPR.

- **Compressions**   Push hard and fast, in the center of the chest for 30 compressions, at a rate of 100 per minute, with compression depth of at least two inches.

- **Airway**   Open the airway using the head-tilt/chin-lift method or use the jaw-thrust procedure if spinal injury is suspected.

- **Breathing**   Give two rescue breaths at a rate of one per second. (CPR mask and gloves are recommended.)

CPR alone is unlikely to restart the heart. The purpose of CPR is to restore partial flow of oxygenated blood from the heart to the brain. This allows a brief opportunity for successful resuscitation without permanent brain damage. Use of an automated external defibrillator (AED) to shock the heart (defibrillation) is usually needed to restore regular heart rhythm.

Abdominal Thrust Procedure

Abdominal thrusts (also known as the Heimlich maneuver) are an emergency first-aid procedure to prevent suffocation. It is used only when there is complete obstruction (blockage) of the airway. Abdominal thrusts are used to dislodge the obstruction and force it upward, out of the throat.

Clutching the throat is the universal sign for choking. In case of choking, ask the person to speak or cough. If the person cannot speak or cough, or if the response is very weak, quickly proceed with abdominal thrusts.

If the person is conscious, follow these steps:

1. Stand behind the person.

2. Slide your arms under the armpits, and wrap them around the person's waist.

3. Make a fist with your hand; place the thumb side against the victim's abdomen, just above the navel and below the ribs. Grasp your fist with your other hand.

4. Quickly thrust inward and upward to force enough air from the lungs to expel the obstruction. Give thrusts with the intent of expelling the obstruction.

5. Repeat. Continue the thrust procedure until the object is dislodged and the person is breathing normally.

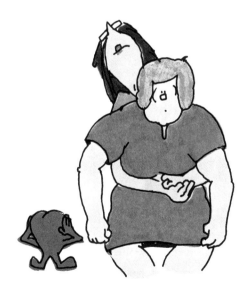

If a person becomes unconscious, begin first aid procedures immediately. Your quick actions and first aid/CPR skills may save a person's life.

1. Call for help.

2. Carefully lower the person to the ground and position face-up on a firm, flat surface.

3. Begin CPR, starting with compressions.

4. Look in the mouth for an object after each set of compressions, before giving rescue breaths.

5. If an object is visible, try to remove it. Be careful not to push the blockage into the throat.

6. Continue CPR. After each set of compressions, check whether the blockage has dislodged and can be removed. Continue CPR until medical help arrives or the victim shows obvious signs of life.

This information is a general overview. Attend a CPR course for detailed training.

Part 5 — Using Protective Devices

Restraints are a last-resort measure that requires a doctor's written order.

Restraints are intended to be protective devices that prevent residents from injuring themselves or others. There is strong emphasis on not using restraints. However, Nursing Assistants need to know how to use restraints when doctors order them as a last-resort measure. Never use restraints unless directed by your supervisor. Legal charges may be filed if restraints are used unnecessarily.

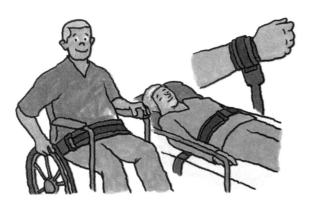

Restraints require a doctor's written order specifying the type of device to be used, length of time, and the purpose for using the device. Restraints are used as a last resort when alternative methods have failed, and they must be used in the least restrictive way possible.

You need to know how to apply restraints properly and safely. Learn to tie knots that can be released quickly in an emergency. Practice quick-release knots until you feel confident with your skills.

Monitor restrained residents frequently, and anticipate their needs. Anyone who is agitated or combative needs to be monitored continuously. Others need to be checked within 30 minutes or less. Careful observations include breathing, circulation, skin irritation, safety, mobility, and comfort.

Restraints add to the risk of pressure ulcers, urinary infection, pneumonia, and other problems. Sometimes restraints reduce independence and social contact, which can contribute to emotional problems such as depression, withdrawal, and agitation.

Lack of movement can weaken muscles, decrease appetite, interrupt sleep patterns, and cause cardiovascular stress. Remove restraints at least every two hours. Allow normal body function for a few minutes before reapplying the restraint. Follow the care plan and facility guidelines.

Applying Restraints

If the doctor orders restraints*, follow the instructions carefully. Restraints can cause serious injuries if they are not applied correctly. Never tie a restraint to the side rail; it might tighten if the rail is raised.

1. Tell the resident why you are applying the device.

2. Tie snugly, without cutting off circulation. Check to be sure you can slip your fingers under the device after tying.

3. Pad the device to protect skin and joints and to avoid discomfort. Position the resident to avoid irritation from knots and buckles.

4. Straighten wrinkled clothing or linen.

5. Make the resident comfortable, and place a call signal and personal items within easy reach.

6. Check the resident within 30 minutes or less to be sure the device has not tightened or slipped with movement. Report any redness or skin irritation.

7. Remove the device within two hours; offer toileting or check pad for dryness, offer fluids, encourage ambulation (if able), check skin condition, and reposition the resident.

8. Allow a few minutes for normal body functioning before you reapply the restraint.

9. Carefully document the use of restraints, and report any problems or concerns immediately.

Be sure you know how to use restraints correctly and safely. Incorrect use can cause serious harm.

*Note that raising the side rails on a resident's bed is a form of restraint. If you have questions or concerns about the side rails, ask your supervisor.

Alternatives to Restraints

Whenever possible, the care team should consider activities that might reduce the need for restraints. Following are suggestions:

- companionship and supervision
- physical and mental activities
- therapeutic touch
- supervised outings
- emotional support
- restorative programs (e.g., strengthening exercises to promote safe ambulation)
- specialized programs for residents with dementia
- music therapy, reminiscence
- programs to allow safe wandering (such as alarms and good supervision)
- mattresses that are ordered for the floor to reduce injuries from falls
- preventive programs to calm aggressive behavior (e.g., approaching residents in a quiet and calm manner, not rushing them).

Follow each resident's plan of care. The plan is based on assessment of the resident. Talk to your supervisor if you have questions or concerns about restraints or protective devices.

Summary

The resident's safety and well-being are the NA's top priorities. The best way to avoid emergencies is to use preventive measures. Emergencies happen. Learn the facility's emergency procedures, and stay current with first aid and CPR training. In case of emergency, stay calm and respond quickly. Never use restraints unless you are directed by your supervisor. Limit the need for restraints by practicing alternatives to restraints.

Review

1. Identify six or more ways to prevent falls.

    _____

    _____

    _____

    _____

    _____

2. How can you prevent accidental poisoning?

    _____

    _____

    _____

    _____

3. List three hazards that cause burns.

    _____

    _____

    _____

    _____

4. How can you help prevent fires?

    _____

    _____

    _____

    _____

5. In case of a catastrophe, what is the top priority?

    _____

    _____

    _____

    _____

    _____

6. When would you use CPR?

    _____

    _____

    _____

    _____

7. Describe the abdominal thrust procedure, and when you would use it.

    _____

    _____

    _____

8. List four or more alternatives to restraints.

    _____

    _____

    _____

    _____

Module 11

Providing Good Nutrition

Everybody needs a variety of foods for good health.

Objectives:

- Identify basic food groups
- Explain the importance of good nutrition
- Recognize conditions that affect eating habits
- Discuss changes in behavior that may relate to improper nutrition
- Explain how to prevent complications from dysphagia

Need-to-Know Words:

- nutrition
- food groups
- therapeutic
- dietician
- diet card
- aspiration
- dysphagia

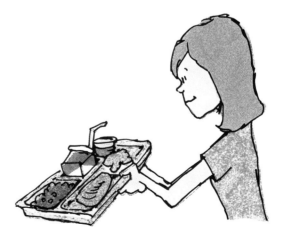

Part 1	Understanding Nutrition

A balanced diet is essential for health and body functioning.

Eating right is vital to each person's physical and emotional well-being. Good nutrition maintains health and body functioning and increases the ability to fight infections. Poor nutrition causes health problems and sometimes relates to behavioral changes.

Unmet nutritional needs can cause the following conditions:

- lack of energy, fatigue
- lack of interest
- irritability, fear, anxiety
- loss of appetite

Elderly people have the same nutritional needs as younger people. However, they usually need fewer calories because they are less active. Eating a variety of foods provides the necessary nutrients for body functioning.

A diet low in fat helps maintain healthy weight. Maintaining healthy weight decreases the risk of high blood pressure, heart disease, stroke, certain cancers, and diabetes.

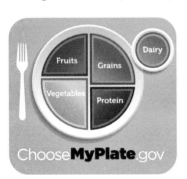

MyPlate was introduced in 2011 (replacing the Food Pyramid) by the United States Department of Agriculture (USDA). MyPlate is a general guide for maintaining a healthy diet. A wealth of information about nutrition is available on the internet at *ChooseMyPlate.gov.*

The information is personalized, focusing on a balance between how much a person eats and how many calories a person burns. Emphasis is on healthy choices, and calorie levels are based on age, gender, and physical activity.

Monitoring body weight helps determine whether an individual's intake needs to be adjusted. An increase in exercise generally allows for an increase in calories.

Following is a brief overview of MyPlate's five food groups plus oils.

- **Vegetables** - promote variety and emphasizes dark green and orange veggies.

- **Fruits** - emphasize variety including fresh, frozen, canned and dried fruit.

- **Grains** - include any food made from wheat, rice, oats, cornmeal, barley, or another cereal grain (e.g., bread, pasta, oatmeal, breakfast cereals).

- **Protein Foods** - include meat, poultry, seafood, eggs, nuts, dry beans and peas.

- **Dairy** - includes fluid milk and foods made from milk that retain calcium content (e.g., yogurt, cheese). Most choices should be fat-free or low-fat.

- **Oils** provide essential nutrients. The USDA includes them as a food pattern (not a food group). Oils are fats that are liquid at room temperature. They come from plants and fish.

Tips for making healthier food choices:
- Make half your plate fruits and vegetables.
- Make at least half your grains whole grains.
- Switch to non-fat (skim) or low-fat (1%) milk.

Examples of suggested healthy diets from MyPlate designed for older adults — exercising less than 30 minutes a day:

Food Group	Female *1600 calories*	Male *2000 calories*
Vegetables	2 cups	2½ cups
Fruits	1½ cups	2 cups
Grains	5 ounces	6 ounces
Protein Foods	5 ounces	5½ ounces
Dairy	3 cups	3 cups

Doctors develop therapeutic (healing) diets for each resident. A dietician specializes in diets and prepares meals according to doctors' orders.

Following are examples of special diets:

- salt restriction
- clear fluids
- mechanical soft
- full fluids
- pureed
- soft
- diabetic
- bland

Observe each resident's normal eating habits to determine whether nutritional needs are being met. Be sensitive to likes and dislikes, and report food preferences to your supervisor. Chart the exact amount of food and fluid the resident eats and drinks. Accurate records are very important for making decisions about the resident's care.

Special eating utensils are available if needed to help residents feed themselves. Training and encouragement are necessary to help residents use special spoons, forks, cups, and plates.

Following are physical and mental conditions that can affect eating habits:

- digestive problems
- medication
- loss of teeth or poorly fitted dentures
- reduced sense of taste
- swallowing difficulty
- inability to eat without assistance
- emotional upsets, depression

Ensure that residents meet their nutritional needs by assisting them whenever they need your help. Nutritious food and beverages are vital for physical and mental well-being.

Part 2 — Serving Food

Make mealtimes enjoyable for the residents.

Dining with others provides an opportunity to socialize. Encourage residents to go to the dining room for meals if possible. For residents who must eat in their rooms, take a few minutes to chat and make mealtime special. Provide assistance as needed, and check care plans to find out whether self-feeding programs have been developed.

Assisting Dependent Residents

Some residents cannot feed themselves and are completely dependent on others to feed them. Always be sensitive to their feelings of helplessness, and remember that it may be frightening or frustrating to be completely dependent on others for basic care.

Choking on food can be a life-threatening emergency. Be sure you know how to perform the abdominal thrust procedure (pages 95-96).

Getting Ready

Wait until you are ready to serve the food before you bring the tray into the room. Follow these guidelines to get ready.

- Position the resident for comfort and safety (sitting upright at 45-90 degrees with the head stabilized).

- Remind the resident to wear dentures if needed.

- Assist as needed with washing hands and face.

- Be familiar with the resident's diet and any restrictions (e.g., calories, sweets, salt).

- If the resident has been incontinent, change the person before serving food.

- Explain how to use special eating utensils, and encourage residents to use adaptive self-feeding devices.

- Understand progressive self-feeding programs, and encourage self-feeding for residents who are able.

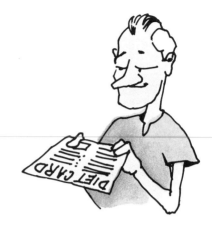

- Check the diet card and compare it with the meal you are serving to be sure it is the correct meal.

- Make sure the tray has the correct food, beverages, silverware, napkins, cup, straw, etc.

- Provide special eating utensils for residents who need them.

- Pick up eating utensils by the handles.

- Keep your fingers out of the food and beverages.

- Assist as needed with pouring drinks and cutting food.

> Always check the resident's diet order card with the meal being served. Serving the wrong meal could cause severe problems.

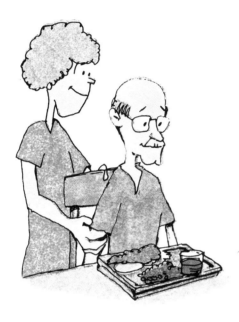

Serving Meals

Follow these guidelines whenever you serve food.

- Wash your hands before and after serving food, and be sure your fingernails are clean.

- Keep your hands away from your face and mouth.

- Be sure your clothing is clean.

- Tie your hair back if it is long.

- Protect any cuts with a waterproof bandage or disposable gloves.

- Check the resident's wrist identification, and ask the resident to tell you his or her name.

  Correct: *"Please tell me your name."*

  Incorrect: *"Are you Mrs. Smith?"*

  (The resident may answer in error.)

Feeding Guidelines

Make mealtimes enjoyable, and be alert to any problems. Follow these guidelines for residents who are not able to feed themselves.

1. Help the resident to an upright position (45-90 degrees).

2. Assist as needed with washing the person's hands.

3. Place the tray where the person can easily see it.

4. Sit beside the person at eye level, and carry on a pleasant conversation.

5. Tell the person what foods are on the tray, and ask what he or she would like to eat first.

6. Feed the food slowly; offer small amounts at a time from the tip of a half-filled spoon.

7. Make sure the person's mouth is empty before offering the next bite of food or sip of beverage.

8. Offer beverages throughout the meal.

9. Allow time to chew and swallow, and watch for signs of gagging or choking.

10. Stop feeding when the resident does not want more or seems tired.

If the resident chokes, remove all food from the mouth and call for help. If the airway is obstructed (the person cannot speak or cough), proceed with the abdominal thrust procedure. (See page 95.)

After the Meal

Remove the tray as soon as the resident has finished eating, and document the amount of food and fluid that was consumed. If the resident did not eat or drink an adequate amount, report it to your supervisor.

Assist as needed with personal cleanliness. Maintain the upright position for 30 minutes after meals to reduce the risk of aspiration (breathing fluid or particles into the lungs).

Snacks

Good nutrition for the elderly may depend on frequent, small meals that provide quality rather than quantity. Check the resident's care plan to find out whether snacks are allowed.

Dysphagia

Dysphagia is difficulty in swallowing. If you observe a resident who has difficulty swallowing, report it to your supervisor immediately.

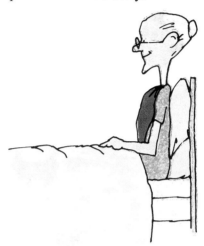

Some foods are more difficult to swallow than others. A person with dysphagia may have difficulty swallowing foods that are pureed or sticky, such as mashed potatoes; thin liquids, such as water; or dry food, such as toast and crackers.

Feeding a resident who has dysphagia requires bolt upright positioning, facing straight ahead. Tilting the head back increases swallowing difficulty and could allow food to enter the lungs. To observe swallowing, watch the Adam's apple rise and fall. Be patient, and do not rush the resident.

Summary

Everyone requires food and fluids for health and survival. MyPlate is a general guide for maintaining a healthy diet. Some residents require special diets. Always check each resident's identification and diet card to ensure that you are serving the right meal to the right person. Make mealtimes enjoyable with pleasant conversation. Avoid rushing the residents, and observe any swallowing difficulties or other problems. Be prepared to do the abdominal thrust procedure if necessary, and report any eating problems to your supervisor.

Review

1. Why is good nutrition important?

2. What is the purpose of MyPlate?

3. List four or more foods from the grain group.

4. Why should you encourage residents to eat in the dining room?

5. What can you do to make mealtime pleasant?

6. List three or more steps to get ready for mealtime.

7. How do you know if you are serving the right meal?

8. What is dysphagia, and how can you prevent problems?

Module 12

Understanding Long-Term Care

Enhance each resident's quality of life.

Need-to-Know Words:
- body systems
- dementia
- reality orientation
- validation
- Alzheimer's disease
- cognitively impaired
- chronic
- cancer
- radiation therapy
- chemotherapy
- anatomy
- physiology
- intravenous
- hyperglycemia
- hypoglycemia
- cardiac arrest
- myocardial infarction
- seizure
- stroke
- TIA

Objectives:

- Recognize emotional and social needs

- Describe behavior management

- Describe body systems and changes related to aging

- Describe confusion and reality orientation

- Describe phases of Alzheimer's disease

- Discuss respiratory disorders

- Recognize side effects of cancer treatment

- Identify symptoms of diabetes

- Discuss steps to take during a seizure

- Describe the symptoms and side effects of a stroke

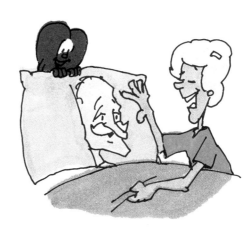

Part 1 Recognizing Emotional and Social Needs

Be sensitive to each resident's needs and concerns.

Growing old affects people physically, psychologically, and socially. Aging brings physical and emotional changes, losses, and different roles. It is difficult for anyone to change from being independent to depending on others for care.

Understand the changes related to growing old. After retirement some people miss the feelings of usefulness, personal satisfaction, and sense of belonging that are related to work. Retirement often means living on less money. Older people may experience loneliness if their families and friends have moved away.

Be sensitive to each resident's needs, and help people adapt to physical and emotional changes. Offer support, reassurance, and encouragement. Provide the same quality of care that you would give your family and loved ones.

Help residents adapt to long-term care. Be a good listener, and ask questions, without prying. Encourage residents to be as self-managing as they are able, and allow them to make choices and decisions whenever possible.

Add variety and interest to each resident's day. Encourage friendships and participation in community activities and social events for residents who are able. Promote interests in appropriate hobbies and activities. Spend extra time with residents who are confined to their beds. Contact with others and loving support is vital to each resident's well-being. Sharing thoughts and feelings with others prevents feelings of isolation. Welcome the resident's family and friends, and allow time and space for private visits when appropriate.

A variety of community resources is available. Find out what is available in your area. Ask your supervisor or the Director of Staff Development for information about local resources.

Managing Behavior

It is normal for anyone who is dependent on others to experience fear and frustration. Fear and frustration can influence behavior and bring out the worst in people. Try to look beyond the behavior to the underlying need for comfort and support.

There will be times when difficult behavior will cause you to feel angry or frustrated. These are normal feelings, but you must control your reactions. Always respond with respect and kindness. Try to understand the reason for the behavior.

There will be times when residents feel angry. Stay calm, and do not take their anger personally. Be patient and understanding, and talk in soothing tones. You may have to deal with temper tantrums, stubbornness, and other difficult behaviors. If the resident becomes combative, get help if necessary. Ask your supervisor about ways to change undesirable behavior through behavior modification.

To increase desirable behavior, use praise or rewards. Following are examples:

- showing respect and making the person feel important
- listening and showing interest
- saying thank you
- smiling and acknowledging accomplishments
- patting the person on the back or giving the person a hug
- offering a special treat

Any corrective action or reward must follow the resident's care plan. If you have any questions or concerns about managing behavior, talk to your supervisor.

Part 2 — Understanding Body Systems

Know the basic body systems and their functions.

To help residents function as normally as possible, Nursing Assistants need a basic understanding of how the body works. You need to know about anatomy (body structure) and physiology (bodily functions).

Each body system has specific functions, but the systems are dependent on each other for function and survival. Problems with one system affect the entire body.

System	Anatomy	Physiology
Circulatory	heart, blood vessels	pumps blood
Digestive	mouth, esophagus, stomach, small and large intestines (bowel), rectum, anus	breaks down food, absorbs nutrients, eliminates waste
Endocrine	glands	regulates metabolism, stores fat for energy, regulates hormones, repairs injured tissue
Integumentary	skin, hair, nails	controls temperature, keeps germs out
Musculoskeletal	bones, muscles, tendons, ligaments	supports and shapes the body, protects organs, enables movement
Nervous	brain, spinal cord, nerves	gathers and sends messages throughout the body
Respiratory	nasal passage, mouth, trachea, lungs	circulates oxygen and removes carbon dioxide (waste product)
Urinary	kidneys, ureters, bladder, urethra	maintains fluid balance, cleanses the blood, eliminates waste

Part 3　　Adapting to Physical Changes

Help people cope with changes.

Nursing Assistants need to understand what happens as a person ages. By understanding the aging process, you will learn to recognize changes and be able to help residents adapt to the changes.

Physical changes are a normal part of aging. Changes are very gradual and vary from person to person. The elderly have greater risk for illness, chronic diseases, and injuries. Inability to function as they could when they were younger impacts people both physically and emotionally.

Learn all you can about age-related disorders. Awareness of problems will help you relate to the people in your care. The following tables will help you understand some effects of aging.

System	Potential Problems	What To Do
Cardiovascular	heart muscle loses strength arteries/veins get narrower, reduce blood flow less oxygen to entire body slower healing	Work with the care team to develop an exercise program. Stimulate circulation with movement. Pace activities. Report tiring from exercises. Elevate legs. Keep extremities warm.
Digestive	less saliva production more difficulty swallowing loss of teeth, harder to chew less taste, less appetite more frequent constipation more indigestion	Encourage fluids. Allow plenty of time to eat. Make sure dentures are in place if used. Encourage frequent toileting and establish bowel movement regularity. Season foods as per diet.
Endocrine	decreased hormone levels less body water so weight loss less ability to handle stress more likely to become ill takes longer to get well	Wash hands often and well. Keep surroundings clean to prevent infection. Reduce stress and avoid schedule changes. Offer encouragement, not criticism.
Musculoskeletal	muscle atrophy, lose strength bones lose density and become brittle joints less flexible gradual height loss	Avoid falls; hip fractures can be deadly. Position and walk as indicated in the care plan. Encourage range-of-motion exercises. Encourage the resident to do as many activities of daily living as possible.

System	Potential Problems	What To Do
Nervous	decreased brain cells less blood to brain forgets recent events	Do not rush the person. Allow time for decisions. Avoid abrupt schedule changes. Encourage thinking, reading, mental exercises.
Reproductive	less ability to get, maintain erection in men menopause in women reduced vaginal lubrication	Recognize that people of all ages are sexual beings. Allow time and privacy for a person's sex life. Be willing to discuss sex openly. Never tease, criticize, or embarrass a person.
Respiratory	lungs lose strength more lung deposits possible harder to breathe increased risk of secretion accumulating in the lungs	Get the person out of bed often. Encourage exercise. Encourage coughing and deep-breathing exercises.
Sensory	reduced vision, hearing decreased taste, smell reduced sense of touch, less likely to feel pain voice muscles lose strength	Encourage use of glasses and hearing aids if needed. Speak slowly and clearly. Listen carefully when the person speaks. Encourage good nutrition even though the food may not taste good to the person.
Integumentary	skin dries, less elastic, tears easily wrinkles, age spots appear skin loses fatty layer so person gets cooler surface blood vessels weaken nails thicken, toughen hair turns grey, falls out skin bruises easily	If bedridden, change positions frequently to help prevent pressure ulcers. Smooth wrinkles from linen. Keep skin clean and dry. Use lotions for moisture. Remove safety hazards. Use extreme care clipping nails. Layer bed covers for warmth. Encourage fluid intake.
Urinary	reduced kidney function less bladder control, incontinence more frequent urination	Encourage daytime drinking of fluids. If the person is incontinent, do not criticize. Follow bladder training program; toilet at least every 2 hours. Position properly for urinating. Keep clean and dry.

Part 4 — Dealing with Confusion

A confused person feels frightened and frustrated.

Some residents need help with mental disabilities as well as physical functions. People who cannot care for themselves require patience and good will to help them cope with situations in which they feel powerless.

Dementia

Dementia is a disorder that impairs a person's mental ability. There are many types of dementias and many causes of confused behavior. Some are reversible, and some are considered irreversible. Dementia is a symptom of brain malfunctioning.

The effect on the person is decreased ability to think clearly, personality changes, and impaired judgment. Dementia affects the person's emotional state and can result in behavioral disturbances. When a resident demonstrates confused behavior, report it.

Making decisions becomes increasingly difficult for people with dementia. Some residents may need to be reminded of activities of daily living such as eating, bathing, dressing, and toileting. Some may wander aimlessly. Sometimes people try to hide their memory loss by making up stories. People with dementia are sometimes confused about time, places, and people. They often remember details from long ago and forget what happened only moments earlier.

More than 100 conditions mimic dementia and can be treated. Following are some treatable conditions that can contribute to mental impairment:

- drug reactions
- anemia
- nutritional deficiencies
- brain tumors
- hydrocephalus
- depression
- head injuries
- thyroid problems

Dementia is usually considered irreversible when it is caused by Alzheimer's disease, strokes, or diseases that affect the nervous system, cardiovascular system, or pulmonary system.

Typically, people with dementia react to their confusion with denial, anger, fear, and grief. They usually resist help and seldom appreciate assistance. Decreased abilities add to mental confusion, and the world becomes a strange and frightening place for people with dementia. The need for supervision and assistance increases as symptoms get worse.

Reality Orientation

Reality orientation is a major part of caring for residents who are confused. Reality orientation is based on repetition. Repetition is useful for all geriatric (older) residents.

- Repeat the person's name often.

- Identify yourself each time you visit.

- Speak slowly and calmly, and use simple words that the resident understands.

- Open the drapes during the day and close them at night.

- Encourage the resident to watch TV and listen to the radio.

- Protect the resident from injury; he or she may not be aware of hazards.

- Avoid rearranging the furniture.

- Give instructions that are easy to follow, and repeat as often as necessary.

- Ask simple questions and allow time for the response.

- Repeat the day, date, and time often, and put calendars and clocks where the resident can easily see them.

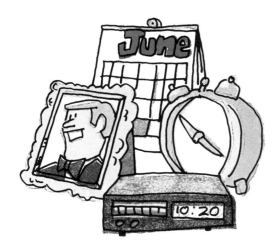

- Discuss familiar people, objects, and events, and keep familiar pictures visible.

- Never rush the resident.

- Encourage socialization; do not isolate.

- Be patient and kind!

Validation, Music, and Reminiscence

Validation therapy is another way to help residents with declining mental ability. You "validate" the person by accepting his or her feelings and "going with the flow." Meet the resident on his or her own terms of reality. For example, if the person is depressed, you would not try to talk the person out of the feelings or say that he or she should not be depressed. Allow the person to experience the feelings.

Appropriate music is another useful form of therapy. It soothes and relaxes residents and brings back memories of people, events, places, and feelings.

Reminiscing about the past is also a form of therapy. Recalling fond memories tends to improve thinking skills and stimulate the senses. Residents may enjoy talking about the past and sharing their wisdom and skills. Taking time to listen gives them a sense of value and belonging.

Alzheimer's Disease

Alzheimer's disease (AD) is a brain disorder with no known cause or cure at this time. It is the most common form of irreversible dementia. More than five million people in the United States are victims of AD, and the number is expected to triple in the next fifty years.

The disease is progressive as it slowly steals the minds of its victims. Early symptoms are gradual and may go unnoticed, including mild mental confusion and mood swings. In the later stages, the person develops severe physical problems and becomes dependent on others for survival.

AD is a terminal illness that affects each resident differently. In general, the disease becomes increasingly worse in three phases, from inability to remember recent events to severe mental decline.

In **phase one (mild),** there may be subtle changes and brief confusion followed by normal behavior. Reactions are slow, judgment is impaired, and decisions may be difficult.

In **phase two (moderate),** the resident functions, but is increasingly forgetful and confused. He or she needs supervision and may need help with activities of daily living (e.g., bathing, toileting, dressing). There may be mood swings and unusual behaviors. The resident becomes increasingly disoriented and cannot remember people and places. It becomes more difficult to speak or understand language, and the attention span becomes shorter.

In **phase three (severe),** the resident becomes totally dependent and needs constant supervision. The resident has difficulty communicating or using good judgment and does not recognize loved ones. The person may lose the most basic abilities including the ability to walk, speak, swallow, control the bowel and bladder, and to follow simple directions. The resident may become bedridden or confined to a wheelchair. Vulnerability to disease and complications increases.

Continue to meet the resident's emotional needs. Accept the person's own reality and validate feelings. For the person who is totally disoriented, validation therapy is less frustrating than reality orientation. Offer your support and understanding, and be considerate of the resident during this difficult time. A gentle hug or touching the person's hand expresses care and affection.

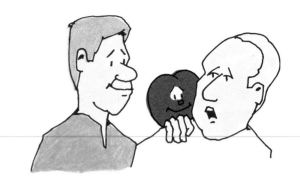

Cognitively Impaired

Cognition is the mental process of learning and acquiring knowledge. People who are cognitively impaired are limited in what they can learn and remember. Some can learn self-care with assistance, and some are totally dependent on others for their care.

Repetition is important when you provide care for someone who is cognitively impaired. Whether you are trying to communicate a skill or an idea, repeat the information step-by-step until the person understands. Always break information into simple pieces.

Use verbal cues. Explain what you are going to do, then talk the person through each step. (For example, feeding steps would be "open your mouth," "insert the food," "chew," and "swallow.")

Learn residents' names. Knowing their names gives the residents a sense that you care about them and makes them feel special.

Treat residents who are cognitively impaired the same as you treat other residents. Make all interactions as normal as possible. Do not talk "baby talk" even when adults act like children.

Part 5 Understanding Chronic Respiratory Disease

Disorders that disrupt air flow can be life-threatening.

Chronic Obstructive Pulmonary Disease (COPD) is a term for permanent lung diseases that interfere with normal breathing and worsen slowly over time. Symptoms include shortness of breath, wheezing, chronic cough, and recurring respiratory infections. Doctors may prescribe medication to make breathing easier. Advanced stages may require oxygen or surgery.

COPD includes chronic bronchitis and emphysema. Most people with COPD have a combination of both conditions. Smoking is considered the most common cause of COPD; quitting prevents further damage. Other causes include exposure to chemicals, air pollution, lung irritants, and second-hand smoke.

Chronic bronchitis includes a long-term cough due to inflammation and mucous in the bronchial tubes (airways). Mucus blocks the tubes, making it hard to breathe.

Emphysema destroys lung tissue over time. The alveoli (air sacs) become stiff and unable to hold enough air. It becomes difficult to get oxygen into the blood and to get carbon dioxide out.

Make sure that residents with progressive lung disease are positioned for easy breathing (e.g., Fowler's position). Breathing may be difficult lying down. Always be alert to breathing difficulties, and report any problems immediately. Respiratory disorders can be life-threatening.

Part 6 — Coping with Cancer

Treatment impacts residents physically and emotionally.

Cancer is a malignant tumor—a growth of abnormal cells that originates in body tissue and organs and spreads to other parts of the body. Cancer comes in many forms. It is not a single disease. The most common cancers occur in the lungs, breast, colon, rectum, prostate, and uterus.

Specific causes of cancer are unknown. Some factors that contribute to cancer have been identified:

- smoking
- radiation
- cancer in the family
- alcohol
- certain chemicals
- certain viruses

Detecting cancer early is important for controlling and treating the disease. The American Cancer Society has identified seven early-warning signs of cancer. **Be alert to these warning signs:**

- change in bowel and bladder habits
- sore that does not heal
- unusual bleeding or discharge
- lump or thickening
- difficulty swallowing or indigestion
- obvious change in a wart or mole
- nagging cough or hoarseness

Three common treatments for cancer are surgery, radiation therapy, and chemotherapy. Surgery involves removing malignant tissue. Radiation destroys localized cancer cells. Chemotherapy uses drugs that travel through the bloodstream to destroy cancer cells anywhere in the body. Treatment depends on the type of tumor, its location, and whether the cancer has spread. Controlling cancer may involve one treatment or a combination of treatments.

Be alert to side effects of cancer treatment. Side effects can affect a person's appetite, energy level, appearance, and physical comfort.

Treatment can cause nausea and vomiting. The resident may lose all interest in food. Provide nutritious foods even if the resident is not hungry. Encourage the resident to eat frequent, small meals. Notify your supervisor if severe nausea and vomiting persist.

Skin becomes easily irritated. Keep the person clean and dry. Avoid pressure, and reposition often. Avoid coarse blankets and talcum powder that can irritate the skin.

A dry mouth is common after treatment. Help keep the resident's mouth clean and moist. Encourage fluids and soft foods. (Check the care plan for any restrictions.) Ice cream, melon, popsicles, and apple juice cool the mouth; hard candy moistens the mouth. Avoid orange juice and other citrus fruits that may irritate the mouth.

Treatment causes fatigue. Reassure the resident that it is normal to tire easily. Encourage plenty of rest, and check on the person often.

Hair loss is common and impacts the person emotionally. Accept the person's temporary baldness, and try to ease feelings of self-consciousness. The person may choose to wear a scarf, wig, or hat.

People with cancer have fears, concerns, and frustrations. Take time to listen when residents or family members want to talk. Protect residents from exposure to infection (e.g., colds, flu); cancer treatment increases the risk of infection.

Report any significant changes and unusual observations to your supervisor (e.g., pain, bleeding, fever, decreased appetite, changes in vital signs, changes in bowel movements). Provide both physical and emotional support for people with cancer.

Part 7 — Caring for People with Diabetes

Diabetes can be controlled through diet, exercise, and medication.

Normally, the pancreas manufactures and secretes insulin, a hormone that regulates blood sugar. Insulin helps the body break down and convert sugars and starches into energy. When the body cannot produce enough insulin or is resistant to insulin, the person develops a chronic disease called diabetes mellitus.

Learn to recognize the symptoms of diabetes:

- excessive thirst
- weight loss
- blurred vision
- frequent urination
- fatigue
- muscle cramps
- skin is easily irritated and slow to heal

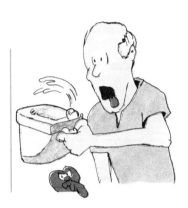

Diabetes is managed with healthy eating, physical activity, and medication (if needed). Careful observation can prevent serious health problems.

- Monitor the resident's food intake, and report any food not consumed.
- Check feet for signs of cuts, wounds, sores, etc., and report any problems to your supervisor.
- Do not trim toenails of diabetics. (Toenails are cut by licensed staff only.)
- Provide a diabetic diet as prescribed.
- Report any changes in level of consciousness. (e.g., unusually drowsy, lethargic, or unconscious).
- Protect against cuts and scrapes. People with diabetes heal slowly and are susceptible to infection; severe infections can result in amputation.
- Keep clothing and bed coverings loose to ensure good circulation.

- Provide good skin care.
- Report any changes in skin color or temperature.
- Report any complaints of pain promptly.

Hyperglycemia is a life-threatening condition caused by too little insulin or too much sugar. The onset is gradual. It occurs when blood sugar levels are high. Elevated blood sugar can cause diabetic coma which can result in death. Hyperglycemia can also lead to kidney failure, blindness, numbness in fingers and toes, stroke, heart attack, and other heart problems.

Early signs of hyperglycemia may include:

- excessive thirst and dry mouth
- increased urination
- drowsiness and fatigue
- headache
- nausea
- abdominal pain

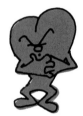

Later signs:

- rapid, heavy breathing
- breath has a fruity scent
- loss of consciousness
- flushed face
- dry skin
- death

Treatment: Insulin is injected by a licensed nurse. Stay with the person, and offer your support. Report anything unusual immediately.

Hypoglycemia is a condition resulting from too much insulin or too little sugar. There is danger of insulin shock when too much insulin has been taken or too little food is consumed. Hypoglycemia comes on very quickly.

Symptoms of hypoglycemia may include:

- headache, dizziness, blurred vision
- weakness, feeling faint
- nervousness, anxiety, trembling
- sudden hunger, craving for sweets
- mood swings, irritability, confusion

- fatigue, insomnia
- heart palpitations
- death

Treatment: Glucose (sugar) is given orally. In severe cases, glucose may be injected intravenously (into the vein) by a licensed nurse.

Part 8   Caring for Heart Disease

Coronary heart disease is the leading cause of death in the United States.

The leading cause of death in the United States is coronary heart disease (CHD). The disease is caused by narrowing of coronary arteries due to a buildup of plaque (fatty material). The most common reason people die suddenly is **cardiac arrest** (sudden, abrupt loss of heart function) due to CHD. Cardiac arrest strikes immediately, without warning. The person loses consciousness and is not breathing normally.

The cardiovascular system is the pumping system of the body. When the blood supply to the heart is reduced, parts of the heart muscle die, resulting in **myocardial infarction (MI)**, also known as a **heart attack**. Heart attacks often start slowly as mild pain or discomfort. Symptoms may come and go.

It is vital to learn the warning signs for cardiac arrest and heart attack. If you suspect any of the symptoms might be present, report it immediately. **Immediate help may save a life!**

Symptoms of a heart attack include the following:

- chest pain that lasts more than a few minutes (e.g., pressure, squeezing, fullness)
- anxiety, sense of impending doom
- shortness of breath
- pain or discomfort in the upper body (e.g., arms, back, neck, jaw)
- dizziness, light-headedness, nausea, breaking out in a cold sweat
- irregular pulse rate, decrease in blood pressure

Decrease any strain on the heart, and make the person comfortable. Follow these guidelines.

- Position the person for easy breathing.
- Elevate the head and chest, and place pillows to support the arms and neck.
- If you must move the person, be gentle.
- Encourage the person to rest.
- Stay with the person, and report any changes in the resident's condition immediately.

Congestive heart failure (CHF) is a condition in which the heart's function as a pump is inadequate. The heart is not able to deliver enough oxygen-rich blood throughout the body.

Common symptoms include:

- fatigue, weakness
- heart palpitations
- shortness of breath
- loss of appetite
- swollen feet and ankles
- a cough

Common conditions that can cause ineffective heart function:

- high blood pressure
- problems of the heart valves
- coronary artery disease
- long-term alcohol abuse

It is critical to follow each resident's care plan. Promptly report any changes you observe.

Part 9   Responding to Seizure Disorders

Residents need to be protected from injury during seizures.

Seizures are caused by uncontrolled electrical activity in the brain. Seizures can happen to anyone. Sometimes they are related to tumors, head injury, fever, chemical imbalance, or stroke. Sometimes no cause can be found to explain why a person has a seizure disorder.

When a person has repeated seizures, the person is said to be suffering from epilepsy (convulsive attacks). The main treatment for epilepsy is medication to strengthen a person's resistance to seizures. It is important that people who have epilepsy take their medication regularly, as prescribed. Epilepsy may be completely controlled with medication, or at least the number of seizures is kept to a minimum.

Some types of seizures include loss of consciousness and intense muscle spasms; others are barely noticeable and are over in seconds. Following are descriptions of common types of seizure disorders.

Generalized absence (petit mal) seizures are characterized by the person looking blank and staring. There may be slight blinking or twitching. This type of seizure lasts for a few seconds, and then normal activity continues.

Complex partial (psychomotor) seizures may start with an "aura" or waning. The person appears confused or distracted and may repeat a series of movements (e.g., plucking at clothes).

Generalized tonic-clonic (grand mal) seizures tend to have a common sequence of events: staring, stiffening of the body (falling to the ground), possible blue color around the mouth, convulsions (jerking movements). Chest muscles tighten and it may appear as if the person has stopped breathing. As the seizure subsides, breathing returns to normal. This type of seizure usually lasts 5-20 minutes.

> Do whatever is necessary to protect the person from injury during a seizure. Do not try to restrain the person. Never pry the mouth open, and do not insert anything into the mouth.

Status epilepticus occurs when a person has repeated tonic-clonic seizures without recovering consciousness. The person may die if not given medical treatment immediately.

Stay calm. Do not hold the person down or try to stop the movements. Stay with the person until the seizure ends naturally.

Follow these guidelines during a seizure.

- Call for help.
- Help the person lie down, and place a pillow under the head.
- If possible, turn the head to one side to prevent choking.
- If the seizure occurs on the floor, move furniture and equipment out of the way.
- If the person is in bed, pad the side rails with blankets or soft foam.

After the seizure, the person will not remember what happened. Offer the person comfort and support, and help the person into bed. Report any seizures to your supervisor, and chart that the seizure was observed and reported.

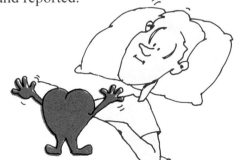

Part 10 — Understanding Strokes

"Brain attacks" result from interruption of blood flow to the brain.

Strokes are "brain attacks" that occur when blood supply to the brain is interrupted by a blood clot, a buildup of plaque, or hemorrhage—damaging or destroying brain tissue. Strokes are also known as cerebrovascular accidents (CVA). Attacks are sudden and can be life-threatening. Like heart attacks, strokes require immediate treatment.

Symptoms come on suddenly and vary in severity. Warning signs may include:

- numbness, tingling, or weakness of the face, arm, or leg, usually on one side of the body
- confusion, trouble speaking or understanding
- impaired vision in one or both eyes
- dizziness, loss of coordination
- sudden severe headache

Many stroke victims lose control of muscles and thought processes. They may know what they want but cannot say or write the words. The person may say "yes" and mean "no."

Hemiparesis is muscular weakness on the affected side. The person is able to move but has no feelings in the limbs, and there is danger of burns, scrapes, and other injuries. **Hemiplegia** is common after a stroke. Paralysis occurs on the side of the body opposite the affected part of the brain (a stroke on the right side of the brain affects the left side of the body).

There are three progressive stages in the recovery phase of stroke patients. Not everyone experiences each stage. **Flaccid** is the first stage; the affected side remains limp and weak. Stage two is **spastic;** the affected side develops some tense muscles, with frequent spasms. Stage three is **recovery;** the affected side regains normal use.

Sometimes a stroke is so severe that the victim may appear to be without thoughts or feelings. On the inside, the person may be struggling to be understood. Whenever you enter the room, greet the person and maintain a positive attitude. Provide comfort and safety, and be patient and supportive.

- Encourage exercise to prevent atrophy and contractures.
- Help the resident reposition often to prevent pressure ulcers.
- Provide good skin care.
- Prevent injury by providing safety measures (e.g., transfer belts, walkers).
- Place daily care items within easy reach and within the resident's visual field.
- Anticipate needs.
- Allow time if communication is slow or difficult.
- Use communication aids (e.g., boards, pads, pencils) if necessary.

Programs such as self-feeding, retraining for activities of daily living, and restorative therapy are developed to help residents regain their independence. Encourage stroke victims to be as self-managing as possible.

A transient ischemic attack (TIA) is considered to be a mini-stroke. A TIA has stroke-like symptoms but is short in duration. Unlike a stroke, the blockage breaks up quickly, dissolves, and does not cause brain tissue to die. TIAs are considered a pre-warning sign that a true stroke may be imminent.

Summary

Help residents adapt to physical and emotional changes related to aging and disease. Learn as much as you can about disorders that affect residents, and be alert to signs and symptoms that could be life-threatening. Help residents function as normally as possible by offering your support, providing quality care, and maintaining a positive attitude.

Review

1. Identify three or more changes related to aging.

_____

_____

_____

_____

2. List five or more ways to increase desirable behavior.

_____

_____

_____

_____

3. How can the NA help a resident who is suffering from dementia?

_____

_____

_____

_____

4. What is COPD?

_____

_____

_____

_____

5. List three or more side effects of cancer treatment.

_____

_____

_____

_____

6. What are the symptoms of diabetes?

_____

_____

_____

_____

7. How would you prevent injury during a seizure?

_____

_____

_____

_____

8. What is CVA?

_____

_____

_____

_____

Module 13

Providing Restorative Care

Encourage residents to be as self-managing as possible.

Objectives:

- Explain the goals of rehabilitation
- Discuss the use and care of assistive devices
- Explain benefits of exercise
- Describe complications of immobility
- Describe activities of daily living
- Describe ROM

Need-to-Know Words

- rehabilitation
- independence
- self-managing
- activities of daily living
- assistive devices
- prosthesis
- vision aids
- hearing aids
- mobility aids
- contractures
- atrophy
- range of motion

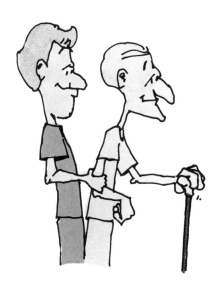

Part 1 — Promoting Independence

Focus on the residents' abilities, not their disabilities.

> The goal of long-term care is to rehabilitate (restore what was lost). Always encourage residents to do as much for themselves as possible. The more you do for them that they can do for themselves, the more you take away their control and contribute to their decline.

Restorative care emphasizes the resident's ability to perform tasks as independently as possible. Restorative care is directed at retraining lost abilities, developing new skills, and preventing complications.

The care team determines what is possible for each resident, establishes realistic goals, and develops a plan of care. The plan encourages independence and promotes the highest level of physical, mental, and emotional wellness. Residents have the right to participate in decisions about their care, and the team encourages them to make personal choices.

Nursing Assistants should encourage and promote improvement at all times. Progress requires guidance, patience, understanding, and sensitivity. Offer support, praise, and encouragement whenever residents are frustrated or discouraged.

The more the residents can do without your assistance, the more you are promoting rehabilitation. You are doing a disservice if you provide care that residents can provide for themselves. One of the biggest challenges in long-term care is helping residents to be independent. Encouraging residents to do things for themselves may take more effort than doing it for them. But it is worth the effort.

Older people have the same basic needs they had when they were younger. They want to feel useful and to keep as much control of their lives as they can.

Activities of Daily Living

Activities of daily living (ADL) are basic tasks of everyday life. Physical and mental disabilities can limit people's abilities to provide their own personal care and mobility. Some residents need help:

- brushing teeth
- eating
- toileting
- dressing
- bathing
- grooming
- walking
- changing positions
- transferring from bed to chair and back

Independence is the goal of restorative care. Encourage residents to be self-managing at every opportunity. For most people, it is a difficult adjustment to depend on others for their basic care.

- Assist only as necessary.
- Break big tasks into smaller tasks.
- Encourage movement and exercise.
- Provide training as needed.
- Help increase strength and ability.
- Encourage use of assistive devices and adaptive equipment as needed.

Family and friends are an important support group for the resident. They provide care and comfort, and they add to the resident's sense of well-being and belonging. Encourage visits, and make visitors feel welcome. Some may want to help care for their loved ones.

Check for any restrictions and follow the guidelines for the facility where you work. If allowed, involve visitors in ADLs (with the resident's approval).

Part 2	**Using Assistive Devices**

Assistive devices help people rely more on themselves and less on others.

Nursing Assistants provide restorative care according to each resident's care plan. The goal is to help residents—physically and psychologically—regain the highest level of functioning.

Assistive devices contribute to a person's independence by helping to regain abilities that were lost due to disease, injuries, surgery, or old age. Sensory aids include glasses and hearing aids. Mobility aids include wheelchairs, canes, walkers, and crutches. Some people wear prostheses. A **prosthesis** is an artificial substitute for a missing body part (arm, leg, breast, eye). Encourage the use of assistive devices as needed.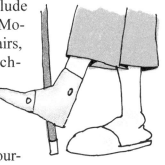

Encourage independence with emphasis on abilities (not disabilities). Assist as needed, and provide emotional support. Proper care and use of assistive devices are important.

- Know the correct way to use a device, and observe whether the resident uses it correctly.

- Inspect the device before and after use to make sure it is in good condition. DO NOT let anyone use a defective device.

- Check for any physical problems related to use (pinching, swelling, rubbing, sore spots).

- Keep the resident's equipment within easy reach.

- Keep the device properly cleaned, and schedule regular maintenance.

- Mark the resident's name in an inconspicuous place for identification including separate items (e.g., removable foot pedals on wheelchairs).

- Encourage residents to help with the care of devices if they are able.

- Observe residents for any problems, and take note of their progress; report your observations.

Devices are available to help residents dress and groom themselves. Dressing aids include zipper pulls, button hooks, long-handled shoe horns, and sock pullers. Grooming aids include combs and brushes with long handles. Provide privacy for dressing and grooming, encourage independence, and assist as needed.

Adaptive products are available to help residents with self-feeding (e.g., plates with built-up edges and/or suction cups to anchor them, cups with special handles, easy-grip silverware). Safety is an important consideration (e.g., whether the resident is able to manage hot beverages).

Vision Aids

Encourage residents to wear glasses if they need them. Eyeglasses are easily misplaced or broken. Follow these guidelines to prevent loss or damage.

- Mark the resident's name on the inside of the frame.

- Make sure there is a case on the night stand for storing glasses. A second case may be needed to carry glasses during the day. Mark each case with the resident's name.

- Provide a neckstrap to keep glasses within easy reach for those who frequently take off their glasses.

- Avoid scratches by cleaning glasses with a soft cloth. (Paper tissues scratch lenses.)
- Check glasses often for loose screws or broken nosepieces.

Contact lenses are an alternative to eyeglasses. Licensed nurses help residents who are unable to care for the lenses themselves. Licensed nurses also provide care for artificial eyes.

Hearing Aids

Some people with hearing loss wear hearing aids. The devices do not correct hearing problems; they make sounds louder. Encourage residents who have hearing aids to wear them whenever possible.

Hearing aids require special care. Be cautious when you handle a hearing aid. Use a table or desk for cleaning the aid or changing batteries to prevent damage if the aid is dropped.

Keep hearing aids dry; water ruins them.

- Remove hearing aids before showering, bathing or swimming.
- If the aid gets wet, dry it immediately with a soft cloth; never use heat.

Keep hearing aids clean.

- Use a soft cloth.
- Never use water, alcohol, cleaning solvents, or oil.
- Remove the aid before using hair spray.

Extend the life of batteries.

- Turn off the hearing aid when it is not in use.
- Disconnect the battery for nighttime storage.
- Remove the battery if the aid will not be used for over 24 hours.
- Check to be sure the battery is working before placing the aid in the resident's ear.

Store hearing aids in a safe place.

- Always use a case for storing the hearing aid, and mark the case with the resident's name.
- Never leave the aid within reach of visiting children.
- Discourage the resident from putting the hearing aid in a pocket (or it may go to the laundry with the clothing).

Hearing Aid Trouble Shooting

Problem	Possible Cause	Action
Doesn't Work	dead battery, plugged earmold	replace battery, clean earmold
Not Loud Enough	low battery, plugged earmold, hearing may have changed	replace battery, clean earmold, have hearing checked
Distorted	low battery	replace battery
Fuzzy	faulty hearing aid	check with supplier
Goes On and Off	bad battery, faulty hearing aid	replace battery, check with supplier
Causes Discomfort	improperly placed, wrong style	check placement, check with supplier

Mobility Aids

Mobility increases independence and decreases complications due to inactivity. Encourage residents to be mobile if they are able. Some residents need mobility aids. The aid must be the right size for the resident, and he or she needs to know how to use the aid correctly.

Be alert to any safety hazards for the residents, and be sure mobility aids are well-maintained. Safety belts are recommended for any chairs with wheels. If equipment is damaged, do not use it. Promptly report any problems or injuries.

Wheelchairs

When using a wheelchair, be sure the resident is properly positioned for comfort and safety. Wheelchairs are equipped with a variety of options. Examples are removable arm rests, heel loops to prevent feet from slipping off, special seat cushions, and footrests. Check wheelchairs often to ensure they are safe.

- Check for loose, worn, or missing parts.
- Check the brakes and report if they do not work properly.
- Keep the chair clean.
- Be sure the chair is properly adjusted for the resident.

Canes and Crutches

A cane is used for balance and support. A cane is usually carried on the person's strong side; it is sometimes used on the weak side for supporting weight. It should be carried on whichever side makes the resident feel more stable.

Observe canes for wear and tear to ensure safe use.

- Check the tips for worn cups.
- Check canes for cracks or loose screws.
- Be sure the resident is using the cane correctly.

Crutches must be fitted correctly based on the person's height. Weight needs to be carried on the hand rests (not on the armpits). Check the person often for friction sores, and check the crutches frequently for safety.

- Check the crutch tips.
- Check the padding for wear.
- Check for loose screws or cracks.

Walkers

Walkers are ordered by a doctor or physical therapist for imbalance or weakness. The type of walker depends on individual needs and ability.

- The standard walker is rigid with four legs. It is used for balance and has suction-cup safety tips.
- The gliding walker is a standard walker except there are wheels on the front legs. The walker can be pushed without having to pick it up. Be alert to safety hazards, and warn residents to be cautious of wheels rolling out from under them.

- The reciprocal walker has a hinged frame and moves forward one side at a time. It has suction-cup safety tips.

A walker needs to be the correct size for the person and checked often for safe use (e.g., no loose screws, no missing or worn parts). To help a resident learn to use a walker, stand behind the person and use a gait belt.

Encourage independence, and praise residents for their efforts and progress with assistive devices. Assist them as needed, and ensure their safety at all times. Observe any difficulties residents have using the equipment, and report any concerns immediately. Careful observation can prevent serious injuries.

Part 3 Assisting with Range of Motion Exercises

Encourage simple exercises to help residents maintain mobility.

Exercise helps maintain bodily functions. It increases blood flow and helps prevent pressure ulcers. Exercise stimulates the bowels and helps prevent constipation. People who exercise are less likely to have urinary infections and kidney stones. Exercise also prevents fluid from collecting in the lungs and causing pneumonia. The benefits of exercise are countless.

Encourage activities and exercises as instructed by your supervisor and specified in each resident's care plan. Prevent complications of immobility by keeping residents as active as possible. Leaving a resident in one position for too long can cause serious complications. Short-term neglect results in long-term problems.

Contractures are a major problem for inactive people. Contractures are caused by shortening or tightening of muscles or tendons, resulting in loss of motion in the joint. Contractures can develop within a few days if joints are not moved through the full range of motion frequently. Following are examples of contractures:

- hip flexion contracture — hips bent, unable to stand straight
- heel cord contracture — toes pointed downward ("foot drop")
- knee flexion contracture — knees bent, unable to straighten
- neck flexion contracture — unable to lift head, rounded back

Other complications of immobility:

- muscle atrophy
- pneumonia
- constipation
- edema
- pressure ulcers
- urinary problems
- osteoporosis
- deep venous thrombosis

Range of motion (ROM) exercises involve moving each joint and muscle through the full range of motion. ROM exercises help to increase the mobility of joints and prevent contractures and atrophy.

Some residents need help with exercises. The care plan will specify the level of assistance each resident needs. Following are common abbreviations for ROM instructions.

PROM	passive range of motion (resident is unable to assist; healthcare worker must move joints for the resident)
AROM	active range of motion (resident can exercise unassisted)
AAROM	active assistive range of motion (resident is able to assist)
UE	upper extremity
LE	lower extremity
RUE	right upper extremity
LUE	left upper extremity
RLE	right lower extremity
LLE	left lower extremity

Guidelines for ROM exercises

To maintain function, flexibility, and strength, residents need to use their muscles and joints. NAs perform ROM exercises as directed by licensed staff and according to each resident's care plan.

Stop immediately if pain or discomfort occurs. Ask the person to tell you if he or she experiences pain during exercise. Watch the resident's face for signs of pain, and stop ROM exercises whenever pain is indicated. Report any pain or problems.

Never exercise a joint that is red or swollen until directed by your supervisor.

- Position the resident in good body alignment for exercising.
- Explain what you are doing and why.
- Do only the exercises that you know how to do, as directed in the care plan.
- Support each limb as you move it gently and smoothly through its normal range.
- Observe any increase or decrease in mobility.
- Never force a joint or move it beyond the person's comfort point.
- Exercise one side completely, and then the other side.

    Generally each exercise is repeated several times, twice a day. (Follow the care plan and facility procedures.)

Terms for ROM exercises:

abduction	moving a body part away from the body
adduction	moving a body part toward the body
extension	straightening a body part
flexion	bending a joint or limb
hyperextension	excessive straightening
dorsal flexion	bending backward
rotation	turning a joint
internal	turning inward
external	turning outward
pronation	turning the joint down
supination	turning the joint up

Encourage residents to perform ROM exercises whenever possible, and train family members to assist if allowed.

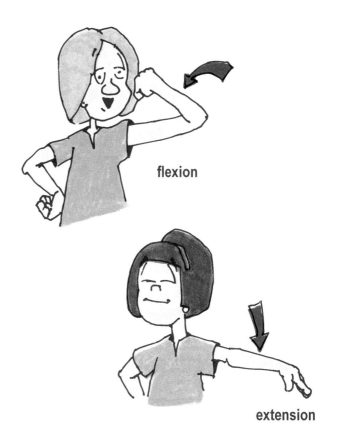

flexion

extension

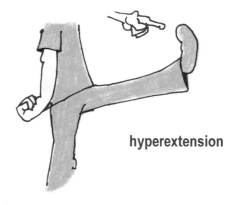

hyperextension

Summary

Restorative care focuses on making residents as independent as possible. Help residents be as self-managing as possible with activities of daily living. Encourage the use of assistive devices for those who need them. Be alert to equipment defects and safety hazards. Help residents maintain strength, flexibility, and function with ROM exercises. Follow each resident's care plan and facility procedures.

Review

1. What are three goals of restorative care?

2. Why should you encourage residents to be self-managing?

3. Describe several activities of daily living.

4. List four or more guidelines for promoting independence.

5. Identify ways to prevent losing or damaging glasses.

6. Describe proper maintenance for hearing aids.

7. Why is mobility important?

8. What is ROM, and why is it important?

Module 14

Managing Information

The care team depends on you for accurate, thorough, and timely reports.

Objectives:

- Explain the importance of careful observation
- Recognize symptoms of abnormal changes
- Explain the importance of detecting problems early
- Discuss the reporting process
- Explain charting procedures
- Discuss the need for accuracy

Need-to-Know Words:
- observe
- timely
- report
- HIPAA
- objective
- subjective
- chart
- document
- care plan
- flow sheets

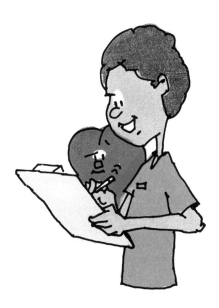

Part 1   Observing, Reporting, and Charting

Carefully observe each resident throughout your daily contacts.

Nursing Assistants need to be alert to problems or changes in each resident's physical or emotional condition. Follow facility procedures for what to report immediately and what to report in writing. Accurate, thorough, and timely records of care and observations of each resident are critical.

All information is confidential, and records must be safely stored when not in use. Some facilities keep handwritten records, and other facilities use computerized systems.

The HIPAA* Privacy Rule provides federal protection for personal health information. All records (written or electronic) are confidential. As a health-team member, it is critical that you understand the facility policies regarding the safekeeping and privacy of all records.

* Health Insurance Portability and Accountability Act

> Everything in the chart is confidential.
> Keeping the information confidential is your responsibility—legally, ethically, and morally.

Observing

Observe each resident throughout your daily contacts. Being a skilled observer helps prevent serious problems and earns the respect of the nursing staff. Being alert to the resident and the environment reduces safety hazards and health problems. Careful observation increases your awareness of each resident's physical, emotional, and social needs.

Learn to recognize signs and symptoms of common diseases and conditions. Detecting problems in their early stages is critical. Trust your instincts. If something seems wrong, report it.

Be alert to emotional changes:
- mood swings, loss of control
- depressed, hopeless, crying, tearful
- angry, difficult, irrational, agitated
- disoriented, confused
- anxious, frightened, pacing, restless

Be alert to physical changes:
- decreased or increased functioning (e.g., pulse, breathing, elimination)
- unconscious, weak, dizzy, drowsy
- shaking, trembling, spasms
- chest pains
- cold, pale, clammy, chills
- hot, burning, sweating, feverish
- nausea, vomiting
- odor
- diarrhea, constipation
- excessive thirst, change in appetite
- change in skin color
- ringing in the ears
- blurred vision
- swelling, edema
- rash, hives, blisters
- choking, coughing, wheezing, sneezing
- shortness of breath
- red or irritated areas, pus, drainage
- change in activity level
- weakness on one side

Reporting

Thorough and accurate reports are made to the nursing staff as often as the resident's condition requires. End-of-shift reports to the oncoming staff provide the information necessary for continued good care. Follow facility procedures.

Objective *(fact)* **reporting** means to report precisely what you see, smell, feel, or hear. Use objective reporting whenever possible.

Examples of objective reporting:

Mrs. Jones's right arm is red, swollen, and warm to the touch.

Mrs. Smith has a persistent cough.

Subjective *(opinion)* **reporting** includes symptoms that the resident can describe (e.g., pain, nausea).

Examples of subjective reporting:

Mrs. Johnson says her stomach aches.

Mr. Adams says he feels dizzy and weak.

Report any new or unusual behavior compared with previous observations. Also report any complaints, pain, or discomfort. If you think something is wrong, report it.

Charting

A chart is the resident's written medical record. NAs are legally responsible for documenting complete and accurate details of all care they provide. The chart is a legal document, and accuracy is very important. Legally, if it is not charted, it is not done.

The chart is a permanent, legal record of care that includes progress notes, physician's orders, medications, treatment and flow sheets, x-ray and lab reports.

Resident care flow sheets detail what needs to be done and include a daily checklist that must be signed when completed. Following are examples of information included in flow sheets.

- *Intake and output* is a record of everything taken by mouth, intravenous feedings, or nasogastric tube, and everything that is eliminated.
- *Tray monitor* is a record of what the resident has eaten.
- *Turning schedule* records positioning.
- *Bowel and bladder retraining* details activities for controlling elimination.
- *Behavior modification* is an action plan for behavior adjustment.

To chart information, complete each blank on the list. If you are unable to complete a task on the flow sheet, initial the appropriate space and circle it. Write an explanation on the back of the page, and report it to your supervisor.

Chart according to facility procedures, and follow these guidelines.

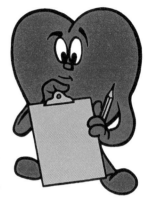

- Be sure the resident's name and room number are on each piece of paper.
- Write clearly and neatly in ink.
- Correct errors by drawing a single line through the error and signing it. Never scribble, erase, or "white-out" a record.
- Chart procedures after completing them; never pre-chart.
- Chart details and time of observations.
- Give only facts, not opinions.
- Be brief without leaving anything out.

Charts are written records of residents' treatments, care, and condition. Accuracy and clarity are critical.

Use the **Tips and Terms Flash Cards** in this book to improve your skills and to learn symptoms and danger signs.

Summary

Nursing Assistants can prevent serious problems by learning to be skilled observers. Be aware of each resident's physical, emotional, and social needs, and always be alert to signs and symptoms that could mean trouble. NAs are responsible for prompt, thorough, and accurate reporting, charting, and documenting of each resident's care.

Review

1. Why is careful observation important?

2. What are three requirements for reports?

3. List five or more physical changes that should be reported.

4. List five or more emotional changes that should be reported.

5. Why is it important to detect problems in the early stages?

6. What should the NA do if something seems wrong?

7. What are flow sheets?

8. Explain the procedure for charting in a resident's record.

Module 15

Dealing with Death and Dying

Provide sensitive and concerned care for residents and their families.

Objectives:

- Define grief
- Explain five stages of grief
- Discuss reactions to death and dying
- Describe care for someone who is dying
- Identify signs of approaching death
- Describe postmortem care

Need-to-Know Words:
- grieving process
- sensitivity
- denial
- anger
- bargaining
- depression
- acceptance
- resignation
- compassion
- postmortem

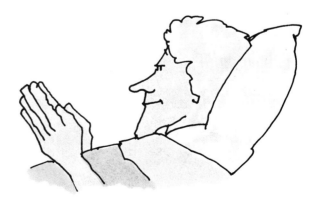

| Part 1 | # Caring for Someone Who is Dying |

Fear is a common reaction to death.

People nearing the end of life need tender care, affection, and comfort. A resident who is dying may depend on you totally for personal care and attention. Tend to the special needs of the resident and significant others with sensitivity and concerned care. Do not allow your fear of death to stop you from being sensitive to a person's needs.

Five stages of grief were identified by phychiatrist Dr. Elisabeth Kübler-Ross in her work with dying patients. The stages apply not only to death, but to any major loss. Not everyone goes through all five stages, nor is there a timetable for the various stages. People may repeat stages in the grieving process.

People who believe they are about to die react in different ways, and the grieving process changes from day to day. Help residents and families through difficult times, and always provide the best care possible.

Denial is the first stage. The dying person is in a state of shock and does not accept what is happening. The person may insist that the doctors have made a mistake or may ignore the facts completely. Sometimes a person is in denial until death occurs. Give people time to adjust. Never force them to face the truth. Listen if they want to talk, but never force conversation.

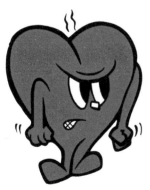

Anger is the second stage. When the person can no longer deny what is happening, it is normal to become angry. The person may strike out with rage and resentment. The person might yell at you, accuse you of poor care, complain about everything, or refuse to do anything you ask. Do not take the attack personally. Try to understand the grieving process and help the person and the family through a very difficult time. The person's family may feel helpless, hopeless, and hurt. Losing a loved one is a very painful experience.

Bargaining is the third stage. The person tries to make deals to postpone death. The person may bargain with God or the doctors, and may try to bargain with you. Listen with a caring attitude, and hold the person's hand for comfort. Never make promises or say, "Things will be all right."

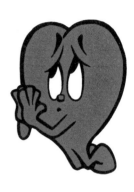

Depression is the fourth stage. As a person begins to accept death, he or she may become very withdrawn. The person may not want to eat or interact with others. The person may cry and need more of your time for comfort and understanding. Be understanding of the person's fears and concerns. Use every opportunity to be reassuring and to enhance the person's self-esteem. Show compassion, and let the person know you care.

Acceptance is the fifth stage. The person is resigned to the fact that death is inevitable. It does not mean that the person wants to die. Provide the same good care for someone who is dying as you would to any other resident. Offer emotional support for the person, family, and loved ones who are overwhelmed with grief and sorrow.

For anyone who is facing death, be there to hold a hand and keep the person from feeling alone. Provide privacy with loved ones. If a clergy member is requested, let your s.upervisor know immediately.

Nursing Assistants help meet the needs—physical, emotional, social, and spiritual—of dying residents.

Death is near when the body begins to shut down and the physical system stops functioning. Dying is a time of crisis, fear, and uncertainty for friends and relatives of the departing person. Provide the best possible care and support.

Allow residents to make choices and decisions whenever possible. Some residents want to be alone. Others may want you to stay nearby or to sit quietly and hold their hands. Some residents may want to talk about their concerns and fears. Be sensitive to individual needs, and provide as much comfort and support as possible. Respect the need for privacy with family and friends, and allow people to die with dignity.

Comfort is key, along with respect for the resident's values, beliefs, and lifestyle. Following are guidelines to care for someone who is dying.

- Keep the call signal within easy reach, and stay nearby.
- Keep the person clean and dry.
- Reposition every hour or two.
- Elevate the head of the bed if the person is short of breath or choking.
- Provide oral care every two hours, and apply lubricant to dry lips.
- Give a back rub if desired.
- Encourage the resident to tell you how he or she prefers to be supported.
- Keep the room well-lighted and ventilated.
- Talk in a normal voice.
- Listen if the person wants to talk, and accept what the person says.
- Provide spiritual support if requested.
- Do not offer false hope.
- Do not say anything you would not want the resident to hear. (The resident may hear you even when unconscious.)

Death may be sudden, without warning. Or it may occur slowly as body processes weaken. Provide care that allows the person to die in peace and with dignity.

Report any physical changes immediately. Signs and symptoms of approaching death may include the following:

- irregular pulse that is rapid and weak
- cold hands and feet
- perspiration (even though the person is cold)
- gurgling sound in the throat
- lack of eye movement, fixed gaze
- breathing that is slow and difficult
- cyanosis (bluish color) of fingertips, toes, lips
- incontinence, urinary retention
- restlessness, agitation, confusion
- nausea, vomiting

After death, the person has the same right to be treated with respect and dignity and the right to privacy as during life. Postmortem (after death) care begins as soon as the person is pronounced dead. Depending upon the regulations and policies where you are employed, you may be asked to provide or assist with postmortem care. Use infection-control precautions. Follow your supervisor's instructions and the procedures of the facility where you work.

Summary

Awareness of the grieving process helps guide you through the emotional experiences that are common for people facing death. Provide the best care possible—physically, emotionally, socially, and spiritually. Be supportive of the resident's family and loved ones. Notify your supervisor immediately if you observe physical changes or signs of approaching death. Follow your supervisor's instructions, and observe facility policies regarding postmortem care.

Review

1. Describe the grieving process.

5. How can you help a dying person who is depressed?

2. What is denial, and how should you react?

6. Describe the acceptance stage.

3. Describe appropriate reactions to anger.

7. Describe care for a dying person.

4. Describe the bargaining stage.

8. List five or more signs of approaching death.

Module 16

Introducing Home Health Care

Help the client stay as healthy and self-managing as possible.

Objectives:

- Define home care
- Explain the role and responsibilities of the Home Health Aide
- Discuss the role of the healthcare team
- Describe special concerns for home care
- Discuss home maintenance and safety issues
- Describe family care

Need-to-Know Words:
- HHA
- client
- home health agency
- resources
- family care
- Medicare

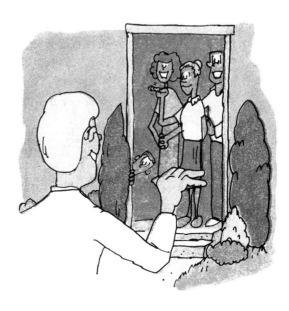

Part 1 Understanding Home Health Care

Be sensitive and flexible to the special needs of the client.

A growing number of people who need assistance with personal care are choosing to stay at home. Home Health Aides (HHA) provide in-home care. This module explains differences and similarities between Nursing Assistants and Home Health Aides.

The same ethical and legal requirements apply wherever you work. Like the NA, the HHA needs to maintain high professional standards and be dedicated to the quality of life for others. In addition, the HHA must be sensitive and flexible to the special needs of home care.

Home Care

Home care enables people to receive quality health care in the comfort and privacy of their own homes. The goal of home care is to help people (clients) to become as healthy and independent as possible. In addition, the HHA helps family members establish routines and carry on normal activities.

Home health agencies employ Home Health Aides as part of a healthcare team. While many home-care agencies provide quality care, those that are Medicare-certified must meet the minimum federal requirements. Medicare-certified agencies represent care standards that are recognized and respected. Clients can use the services of a Medicare-certified agency regardless of how they pay.

Home Health Aides, like Nursing Assistants, work under the supervision of nurses to carry out care plans for clients. Unlike the NA, the HHA works independently in the home and does not have day-to-day supervision. For this reason, Home Health Aides need to be especially mature and reliable. HHAs must be able to work alone, get along with the client and the family, and be dependable.

The HHA may go to the same home every day or may visit several clients on the same day. Duties vary depending on the needs of each client. In addition to personal care, duties may include light housekeeping, shopping, preparing meals, doing laundry, driving the client to and from appointments, and other activities.

The HHA needs to have all the practical and clinical skills of the NA. However, working in a home presents concerns and challenges for the HHA that the NA does not face:

- planning, prioritizing, and organizing the workload
- providing safety and security (e.g., locking doors and windows)
- preventing the spread of infection in a home setting
- making wise decisions when help is not readily available
- performing activities of daily living in a home setting
- being creative
- handling complaints and conflict

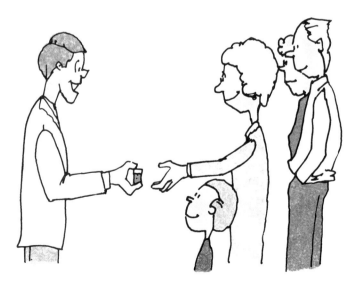

Ability to adapt to home conditions is vital. For example, physical strength is very important since the HHA works alone. Other staff members are not available to assist with lifting and transferring.

Additional concerns for the HHA include:

- home maintenance and safety

- meal preparation, food handling, and storage

- family care and changing needs

- special needs of the client

Careful observation and documentation are very important in the home setting. Medicare requires accurate and detailed reports. Check with the agency for specific requirements.

Certification

Certification is required for Home Health Aides employed by Medicare-certified agencies. Federal regulations require a minimum of 75 hours of training, including 16 hours of classroom instruction, before beginning supervised, practical training.

Certification requires a passing score on tests for practical and clinical skills. In most states the certification requirements for Home Health Aides and Nursing Assistants are the same. Find out what the licensing and certification requirements are for the state where you work.

Client Rights

The HHA must protect and uphold the client's rights. These rights are similar to the rights of residents in long-term care facilities, but there are important differences. Obtain an official copy of home-care rights to understand the differences.

The Care Team

The HHA, like the NA, is part of a team of caregivers. The HHA works under the supervision of a nurse. The supervising nurse visits the client's home at least once a month to be sure that the care plan is working.

Generally, the HHA works with one or two professionals as part of the care team. Team members may be doctors, nurses, nutritionists, physical and occupational therapists, social workers, speech pathologists, or respiratory therapists. The most important members of the team are the client and the client's family. Their involvement and cooperation are vital.

Good communication skills are very important. An HHA must be able to convey information and ideas efficiently and effectively. The care team needs accurate and timely reports about care, progress, and any problems.

An HHA must also be able to communicate well with the client and family. He or she spends more time with them than any other member of the care team.

The alert HHA is the first to notice changes in the client's mood, behavior, and health. Changes in the family can affect the well-being of the client (e.g., unemployment, arguments, or illness).

The HHA needs to be flexible and to have a positive attitude. Everything you do helps the client to maintain independence and to stay at home for as long as possible.

Part 2   Maintaining a Healthy and Safe Home

Keep the home safe and clean for the client.

Before home care service begins, the supervising nurse visits the home to determine the needs of the client. The supervising nurse also checks the home for possible safety hazards. This visit is called a professional assessment.

The assessment determines the plan of care and the HHA's role in the plan. The care plan helps both the HHA and the family understand the HHA's responsibilities. HHAs are only assigned tasks for which they have both training and experience.

A healthy home is important for the client's well-being. You need to know good home maintenance skills and be prepared to teach the skills to the family. Every family has its own ideas about how a household should be managed. The HHA needs to be sensitive to these differences. Never perform any tasks that are not acceptable to the client and family.

Infection Prevention and Control

Pay special attention to procedures that protect the client, the family, and yourself from infections. Hand washing is the most important preventive measure for infection control.

Clean, disinfect, or sterilize care equipment. Be aware of common household items that can spread infection (e.g., sponges, dishcloths, eating utensils, soiled laundry, door knobs, tissues).

Ask the client and family members to cover their noses and mouths with tissues when they sneeze or cough, and encourage hand washing. Dispose of tissues in a covered container.

> Wear gloves at all times when handling blood, body fluids, or needles. Always use precautions to protect yourself, the client, and family members.

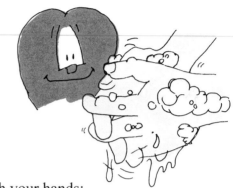

Wash your hands:

- before and after each contact with the client
- before and after eating
- after using the bathroom
- after handling garbage
- after sneezing or coughing

All body waste must be disposed of safely. Liquid waste should be poured into a covered container and taken to the bathroom. Pour the liquid into the toilet bowl. Close the lid, and flush. Clean any spills with a disinfecting cleanser.

Dispose of solid waste in a heavy plastic bag with closures and take the bag to the outside garbage immediately. If a plastic bag is not available, use a paper bag or newspaper. Check that the waste is thoroughly wrapped, with no leakage.

Remove soiled linen from the bed immediately and launder in hot water and strong detergent. If linen is severely soiled or stained with wastes it may have to be discarded.

Dispose of needles in appropriate disposal containers. Be aware that items placed outside for garbage pickup can put others at risk if the garbage is tipped over or gone through. Check with the agency for correct disposal procedures.

Cleaning

The HHA keeps the home healthy by making sure it stays clean. The floors and surfaces of the home need to cleaned regularly. Garbage should be removed daily, and garbage pails need to be washed.

The bathroom needs special attention because of increased risk of accidents and germs. Walls, floors, counter tops, toilets, tubs, showers and sinks must be thoroughly scrubbed with a disinfecting cleanser. Floors should be kept clean and dry, and use nonskid rugs to prevent falls. Encourage clients and family members to hang up wet towels or take them to the laundry room. Remind children that flushing the toilet, rinsing the sink, and washing their hands is part of good personal hygiene.

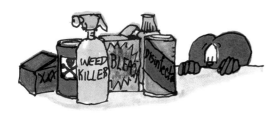

Cleaning products should be kept in a safe place. Read the labels on all household chemicals. Never mix products together because the results can be dangerous.

Always wear disposable gloves when handling chemicals or cleaning surfaces that could be contaminated with bacteria or bodily fluids. Wash your hands before and after all household chores, even if you wear gloves.

Home Safety

The HHA is responsible for maintaining the safety of the client's immediate living area. You must also be aware of any safety hazards within the home. The agency's assessment determines your role in maintaining home safety and the need for safety equipment, (e.g., grab bars, raised toilet seats, bedside commodes, and other devices.)

Simple safety precautions can prevent accidents and injuries. Follow basic safety guidelines.

- Plan an emergency exit and an alternate plan in case of fire or other disaster.
- Provide proper and adequate lighting throughout the house, especially in hallways and stairways.
- Be sure smoke detectors are properly located and working.
- Keep space heaters in good repair and away from low-hanging drapes or other combustible materials.

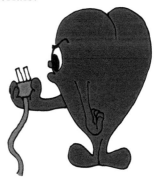

- Keep electrical cords in good repair and out of the flow of foot traffic.
- Keep electrical appliances unplugged when not in use.
- Keep medications labeled and stored securely.
- Use handrails on stairways, in the bath or shower, and other locations where balance may be a problem.

Be prepared in case of an emergency. Follow agency procedures and keep emergency phone numbers readily available by the phone:

- poison center
- fire department
- police
- ambulance

- the agency's number
- client's doctors
- client's family and friends (day and evening numbers)

* See Flash Cards for Emergency Information Card

Kitchen Safety

Pay special attention to kitchen safety and proper food handling. Follow these basic guidelines for kitchen safety.

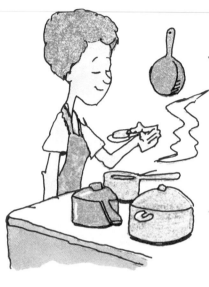

- Always turn off the stove when not in use.
- Never wear long, loose-sleeved clothing while cooking over a hot burner. (Sleeves can catch fire easily.)
- Turn the handles of pots toward the back of the stove when cooking.
- Stay in the cooking area whenever the stove is on high heat.
- Wipe up any spills on the floor immediately to avoid accidents.
- Do not use glasses or dishes that are cracked, chipped, or have jagged edges.

Food Handling

Proper handling of food prevents problems. Follow these guidelines whenever you handle food.

- Wash your hands before and after handling food.
- Wear gloves if you have any cuts or abrasions on your hands.
- Be sure that the area where you prepare food is clean and dry and that all kitchen utensils have been washed thoroughly.
- Wash all vegetables and fruits thoroughly.
- Be sure that all meat is thoroughly cooked.
- Cover and refrigerate leftovers promptly. If the food is warm, put it in the refrigerator before it cools.

Food Storage

Proper food storage ensures freshness and safety. Follow these guidelines.

- Buy only the amount of food that can be stored properly.
- Be sure the refrigerator works properly and the temperature control is set correctly.
- Cover dry foods such as flour and sugar.
- Throw out any foods that are past the expiration date.
- Keep storage areas clean and dry.
- Check the food storage area regularly for insects or rodents.

Part 3 — Tending to Special Needs

Aging brings changes that need special consideration.

The services provided by the HHA can help elderly clients remain in their homes and function independently. For clients returning home from long-term care facilities, the HHA helps with activities of daily living and adjustments in health and lifestyle. The HHA also helps protect the elderly from abuse or neglect in the home.

People age in different ways and at their own pace. Special considerations for the elderly include physical and mental health, diet, and emotional well-being.

Physical Health

Poor circulation can contribute to an older person's need for warm clothing and warmer room temperatures. Older people are especially at risk during cold winter months. Body temperatures can drop rapidly when exposed to cold temperatures.

Many older people on limited incomes try to conserve by keeping their thermostats too low. Check that the thermostats are set properly. Encourage layers of clothing to provide the best insulation.

Dressing and undressing may tire an elderly person. Check that clothing is easy to remove. For example, velcro can often be substituted for zippers. Simple changes in clothing and environment can help clients feel more comfortable. Assist with dressing and undressing as needed.

Balance may be affected. Railings and assistive devices (e.g., canes, walkers) may be recommended by the supervising nurse or physician. Follow the client's care plan for specific instructions about activity.

Falls are more likely to occur if the client is dizzy from rising too quickly. Encourage the client to pause after rising until he or she feels stable.

Offer assistance as needed in moving the client from bed to chair, chair to standing position, and walking. Clients with heart conditions need to be especially careful to move safely and steadily. Your attention and quick response to any loss of balance help the client feel secure.

Vision and hearing may be impaired. Encourage the use and maintenance of assistive devices. (e.g., hearing aids and glasses).

Help the visually-impaired client by keeping personal items in familiar places. Do not move furniture from its usual location. Keep traffic areas in the home uncluttered. Organize clothes in closets and drawers for easy access. List important phone numbers and

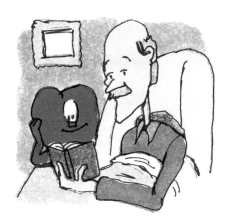

other information in bold, easy-to-read print in a convenient location.

For the hearing-impaired client, speak slowly and clearly. Do not shout. Look the client in the eyes while speaking. Include the client in family discussions.

Self-care should be encouraged. Remember, you are in the home to help the client stay as healthy and self-managing as possible. Allow time for the client to do any tasks that he or she is capable of doing. Speed is not important, but the client's confidence and self-esteem are very important.

Medications

The HHA does not dispense medications but documents whether the client takes medication as prescribed. If the client refuses to take medication or takes more than the prescribed amount, report it immediately.

Report any side-effects of medications:

- diarrhea
- nausea or vomiting
- rash or hives
- headache
- confusion or agitation
- dizziness

All medications must be properly labeled and stored. Note whether refrigeration is required, and note whether medications are to be taken on an empty stomach or with food. Keep all medications out of the reach of children. Take extra precautions with medications when dealing with clients who are confused, forgetful, or have impaired vision.

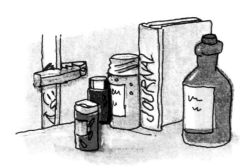

Oxygen

The HHA does not administer oxygen. However, you must understand and report use of oxygen in the home. Teach the client and family members safety rules regarding the use of oxygen. Do not allow smoking, burning candles, or gas heaters near the oxygen room. Post "No Smoking" signs to remind visitors and family members not to smoke. Store oxygen tanks in a cool, secure area when not in use.

Diet

Good nutrition plays an important role in protecting and maintaining health. Basic knowledge of good nutrition is part of the HHA's training. The care plan includes information about the client's diet. Follow the care plan carefully. Serve food at the proper temperature, and arrange food attractively on the tray. Encourage clients to feed themselves if they are able.

It is important for the older client to receive nutritious and regular meals. Without proper nutrition, an elderly person may not have the strength to resist disease. Older people living alone may skip meals out of loneliness or the feeling that it is too much trouble to cook for themselves. Mealtime should be an enjoyable and relaxing part of the daily routine.

Whenever possible, involve family members in sharing time and conversation with the client during meals.

Be flexible with the eating patterns of your clients. Some people do well with several small meals throughout the day. Others may prefer to eat large meals in the middle of the day with light snacks in the morning and evening. Follow the care plan, and notify the supervising nurse of changes or complications in eating patterns.

Mental Health

Mental changes related to aging may cause irritability, disorientation, and memory lapses. Do not assume that changes in an older person's behavior or mood are natural signs of aging. Observe, document, and report all changes as they occur.

Clients suffering from memory loss may forget day-to-day information (e.g. doctor appointments or when you are scheduled to be in the home). Help them to remember by marking calendars and posting reminders in appropriate places. Label cupboards and drawers with the contents to help them find things. Keep personal mementos, such as photographs and letters nearby to help trigger memory and orient the client to the surroundings.

Forgetfulness may require you to repeat the same information several times. Be patient and understanding of the client's need for repetition. The client may be irritable. Irritability is often a sign of depression. Encourage the client to talk about feelings, and promote activities to prevent depression. Suggest hobbies that help the client to become more aware of the outside world (e.g., birdwatching, gardening, caring for a pet). Adapt activities to the client's abilities, interests, and living conditions. Encourage family members to participate in activities with the client.

Observe and report any changes in the client's appetite, sleeping patterns, or mood. Pay close attention to expressions of sadness, loneliness, and hopelessness. Take any talk of suicide seriously, and advise your supervisor immediately.

Part 4 — Caring for the Family

Provide comfort, support, and a sense of order.

The HHA helps establish a routine and brings order to a family in crisis. The role of the HHA varies from family to family based on the nature of the problem, the number of children in the home, and availability of other help.

Remember that you are in the home to offer comfort, support, and a sense of order to the family. Listen to concerns, but do not take sides. Treat each family member as an individual. Respect the need for privacy as well as companionship. Encourage the adults in the family to remain as active as possible in the lives of their children. Work towards the future health and independence of the family.

If you observe significant changes or problems, tell your supervisor. For example, report violence or serious arguments, illnesses, suspected drug or alcohol abuse, layoff or unemployment.

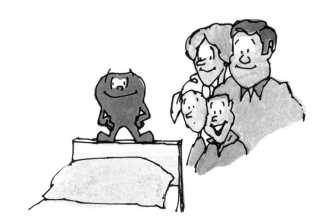

Understanding personality development at various stages will give you important insights into life changes and appropriate care for family members. The chart below is based on **Erickson's Eight Stages of Life.**

Stage	Age	Personality Development	Significant Others
Infant	birth-1 year	learning to trust	mother and/or primary care provider
Toddler:	1-3 years	developing autonomy	parents and primary care providers
Early childhood	3-5 years	recognizing self as family member (initiative)	family, close relatives, and friends
Mid-childhood	6-11 years	demonstrating physical and mental abilities (industry)	relatives, neighbors, school friends
Adolescence	12-15 years	establishing identity	close friends, peers, role models
Young adult	18-40 years	establishing intimacy	marriage partner, family
Middle years	40-65 years	achieving goals	expanded family, work relationships
Older years:	65+ years	satisfying ego, integrity	family and friends who provide a sense of usefulness

Child Care

When a parent is ill or unable to provide necessary care for the children, the HHA establishes a sense of "normal" for the children's daily routine. Children need good food, rest, and play. They also need to feel safe, secure, and capable.

Assure the children that you are there to help. Involve them in basic chores like setting the table, making beds, and choosing clothes to wear. Make as few changes as possible to their daily routine. Change is always stressful, and the family you are helping is already under stress.

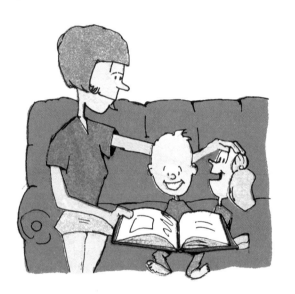

The most common reaction to stress is fear. Common emotional responses to fear include:

- withdrawal, wanting to be alone
- aggression, anger, anxiety, bullying
- sadness, depression, hopelessness

Children express fear in a variety of ways. Common expressions of fear in children include:

- fear of the dark, nightmares
- bedwetting or changes in toileting
- anger and rebellion (e.g., not wanting to go to school, to bed, or to follow any other routine)
- tattling or jealousy of other children in the family
- whining
- clinging

Help children through this difficult time. You can help calm their fears by listening to their concerns. Praise their accomplishments, and always be patient and kind to them.

Part 5 — Finding Resources

Recreation and leisure activities promote well-being.

Social and recreational activities are good therapy and break the monotony of everyday living. Learn which hobbies, interests, and activities your clients prefer. Allow clients to choose activities, but be sure the chosen activities do not conflict with care plans or expose anyone to unnecessary risk.

Be informed about opportunities and resources that are available for your clients. A variety of services are available for senior citizens.

Get information about any programs that fit the needs and interests of your clients. Take advantage of senior discounts at local stores, pharmacies, restaurants, movie theaters, etc. If clients are able to travel, check on special fares for seniors. Find out if the local college offers senior citizen classes at reduced rates. Before beginning any new activities, always check with the agency first.

Community resources are available for the elderly. Find out what services are available in your community. Information is readily available in local newspapers, at local senior centers, on local television channels, or from other seniors. The Internet is an excellent resource for general information about the elderly.

Following are examples of community resources:

- adult protective services (state, social, and health departments)
- area transit services
- consumer protection (state attorney general's office)
- crisis hotline
- food bank and meals on wheels
- hospice
- senior/community centers
- United Way
- visiting nurses association
- YMCA/YWCA
- local support groups

National organizations also provide excellent information. Some organizations have local and regional offices. Following are national organizations that provide excellent information:

Alzheimer's Association
800-272-3900; alz.org

Alzheimer's Foundation
866-232-8484; alzfdn.org

American Association of Retired Persons (AARP)
888-687-2277; aarp.org

American Cancer Society
800-227-2345; cancer.org

American Diabetes Association
800-342-2383; diabetes.org

American Heart Association
800-242-8721; heart.org

American Society on Aging
800-537-9728; asaging.org

American Stroke Association
800-242-8721; strokeassociation.org

Center for Disease Control (CDC)
800-232-4636; cdc.gov

National Association for Aging & Disabilities
202-898-2578; nasuad.org

National Association for Home Care & Hospice
202-547-7424; nahc.org

National Hospice Organization
800-658-8898; caringinfo.org

National Institute on Aging
Information Center
800-222-2225; nia.nih.gov

Eldercare Locator is a national system that connects people with local information sources. The toll-free number for Eldercare Locator is 800-677-1116; eldercare.gov.

Summary

The goal of home care is to keep clients as healthy and independent as possible in the comfort of their homes. The HHA needs to be sensitive and flexible to the needs of the client and the family. The HHA is part of a care team and works under the supervision of a licensed nurse. The same high standards apply to HHAs and NAs including infection control, clean surroundings, safety, upholding client rights, and tending to special needs.

Review

1. What is the purpose of home care?

_____

_____

_____

_____

2. List five or more special concerns for the HHA.

_____

_____

_____

_____

3. List six or more safety precautions in the home.

_____

_____

_____

_____

4. Describe proper food handling and why it is important.

_____

_____

_____

_____

5. Identify three or more ways to control infection in the home.

_____

_____

_____

_____

6. Describe three or more physical considerations for elderly clients.

_____

_____

_____

_____

7. How can you promote the client's mental health?

_____

_____

_____

_____

8. What is the HHA's basic role in family care?

_____

_____

_____

_____

Preparing for the Certification Exam

Learn by reading, writing, and practicing all skills required for certification.

To become a Certified Nursing Assistant, the candidate must complete a state-approved training program and pass the Nursing Assistant competency examination. The exam includes both a written test and a hands-on skills test in a clinical setting. The candidate must be able to pass the written test and to demonstrate the ability to provide quality hands-on care.

Following is a general overview of the knowledge required for both the written exam and the clinical skills test.

❑ Providing routine care
Examples: vital signs, toileting/bedpans, skin care, activities of daily living

❑ Providing specialized care
Examples: incontinence, catheter care, memory loss, paralysis, death and dying

❑ Understanding the role, duties and responsibilities of Nursing Assistants
Examples: care plans, facility procedures, reporting (including abuse and neglect), getting along with others, managing self-control

❑ Recognizing and handling emergency situations
Examples: heart attack, choking, seizures, chest pain, diabetes, falls

❑ Maintaining health
Examples: infection prevention/control, range of motion exercises, positioning, body alignment, ambulating, hydration, assistive devices

❑ Managing information
Examples: confidentiality, observing, reporting, charting procedures

❑ Promoting self-care
Examples: assisting only as needed, encouraging the residents to do as much as possible, praising accomplishments

❑ Promoting safety
Examples: preventing accidents, reporting problems and concerns, knowing emergency and first aid procedures

❑ Understanding age-related physical changes
Examples: effect of aging on the skin, heart, digestive system

❑ Recognizing psycho-social needs of the elderly
Examples: welcoming visitors, offering support, listening, encouraging friendships, offering choices, promoting hobbies, enhancing self-esteem

❑ Maintaining the resident's environment
Examples: keeping the call light/signal within easy reach, answering the signal promptly, keeping the room tidy and safe, adjusting temperature and ventilation

Clinical Skills

Candidates will be assigned several *direct* skills for the clinical test and will be evaluated on their performance. Read through the list of skills and check off the ones you feel confident you can perform. Work on those you leave unchecked. If you have questions or concerns, discuss them with your trainer.

- ❑ Ambulating
- ❑ Bathing/bedbaths
- ❑ Bed making—occupied and unoccupied
- ❑ Body mechanics
- ❑ Call light/signal
- ❑ Catheter care
- ❑ Communication skills
- ❑ Confidentiality
- ❑ Denture care—cleaning and storing
- ❑ Dressing and undressing (includes elastic stockings)
- ❑ Equipment/supplies disposal
- ❑ Feeding
- ❑ Foot care
- ❑ Gait/transfer belts
- ❑ Gloves and gowns
- ❑ Grooming
- ❑ Hand washing
- ❑ Height and weight measurements
- ❑ Intake and output measurements
- ❑ Medical asepsis
- ❑ Mouth care/brushing and cleaning

- ❑ Nail care
- ❑ Perineal care
- ❑ Positioning
- ❑ Precautions, infection prevention/control
- ❑ Pulse
- ❑ Range of motion exercises
- ❑ Reporting and recording
- ❑ Respiration
- ❑ Restraints and alternatives
- ❑ Serving food
- ❑ Toileting/bedpans
- ❑ Transferring/moving
- ❑ Vital signs—temperature, pulse, respiration, blood pressure
- ❑ Weighing and measuring

Indirect skills will be evaluated throughout the hands-on test.

- ❑ Being alert to safety issues
- ❑ Being courteous and helpful
- ❑ Explaining to the resident what you are going to do
- ❑ Identifying the resident and greeting by name
- ❑ Knocking before entering a resident's room
- ❑ Protecting resident rights
- ❑ Providing comfort
- ❑ Providing privacy
- ❑ Using good communication skills

Practice Test

Test your knowledge of NA basics.

Read, write, and review information in this book. Then use the practice test to check your knowledge. The practice test has 60 multiple-choice questions and 15 true/false questions.

Multiple choice: Circle the letter on the left side of the correct answer.

Sample Question

The MOST important way to prevent germs from spreading is to:

ⓐ wash your hands before and after contact with each person in your care

b. drink plenty of fluids

c. avoid any unnecessary contact with people in your care

d. confine people in your care to their rooms

The correct answer is: "wash your hands before and after contact with each person in your care." Circle the letter "a" next to the correct answer.

True/False: Circle T if the statement is true or F if the statement is false.

Sample Question

Ⓣ F **NAs are important members of care teams.**

The statement is true. Circle the letter "T".

Now you are ready to begin the practice test. Read each question carefully before marking the answer. If you are not sure, mark the answer you think is correct.

Multiple Choice

1. **The MOST important member of the care teams is:**
   a. the doctor
   b. the nurse
   c. the resident
   d. the social worker

2. **Keeping information about residents confidential:**
   a. is not important
   b. is fairly important
   c. applies only to medical records
   d. is a legal responsibility

3. **If you are unable to work, it is MOST important to:**
   a. inform your supervisor when you are fit to return
   b. inform your supervisor at the earliest opportunity that you are unable to work
   c. call your supervisor when you are ready to return to work
   d. send a note to your supervisor

4. **Nursing Assistants report to:**
   a. doctor
   b. director of nursing staff
   c. activities director
   d. licensed nurse

5. **Upholding resident rights:**
   a. is a matter of choice
   b. is a legal requirement
   c. is not an NA's responsibility
   d. applies only if a resident complains

6. **Learn about individual beliefs so you can:**
   a. avoid offending someone
   b. argue about differences of opinion
   c. tease residents about their beliefs
   d. defend your own beliefs

7. **If you think a resident has been abused:**
   a. tell the abuser to stop
   b. keep quiet
   c. report the abuse
   d. wait to see if it happens again

8. **Difficult behavior may be the result of:**
   a. a need for comfort and understanding
   b. old age
   c. stubbornness
   d. bad manners

9. **The NA should deal with sexuality:**
   a. with disgust and disapproval
   b. by taking away the right to privacy
   c. by scolding the residents
   d. in a mature and professional manner

10. **Whenever you feel angry or frustrated:**
    a. try to understand your feelings
    b. stomp out of the room
    c. tell the residents it's their fault
    d. let the residents know you are angry

11. **Whenever verbal and nonverbal impressions are mixed:**
    a. words speak louder than actions
    b. actions speak louder than words
    c. words and actions have the same impact
    d. there is no message

12. **If your supervisor corrects a procedure:**
    a. get defensive
    b. make an excuse
    c. learn from your mistake
    d. blame someone else

13. **If a person is visually impaired, you would:**
    a. scold the person for not wearing glasses
    b. identify yourself whenever you enter the room
    c. discourage the person from being independent
    d. avoid talking to the person

14. **If a person is hearing impaired:**
    a. get the person's attention before talking
    b. scold the person for not wearing a hearing aid
    c. shout
    d. avoid talking to the person

15. **When lifting, it is correct to:**
    a. bend at the waist
    b. keep your back straight
    c. keep your knees straight
    d. keep your feet close together

16. **The primary concern when moving a person is to:**
    a. hurry
    b. keep the person happy
    c. use the muscles in your back for lifting
    d. provide safety

17. Changing positions every hour or two:
a. prevents serious health problems
b. keeps residents awake
c. gives NAs something to do
d. is unimportant

18. Decubitus ulcers are:
a. digestive problems
b. pressure ulcers
c. hiccups
d. a contagious disease

19. Use Universal / Standard Precautions for:
a. lifting procedures
b. pulse
c. ambulating
d. blood and body fluids

20. The MOST important measure to prevent the spread of infection is:
a. fresh air
b. clean clothing
c. hand washing
d. isolation

21. Wear disposable gloves whenever:
a. your hands are cold
b. your hands are dirty
c. you have a cold
d. you might be exposed to blood or body fluids

22. Wearing gloves reduces:
a. the spread of infection
b. pathogens
c. non-pathogens
d. puncture wounds

23. Medical asepsis:
a. decreases pathogens
b. increases pathogens
c. is a medication
d. should be reported

24. Germs are most commonly found:
a. in moist, warm areas
b. in dry areas
c. in cold areas
d. in hot areas

25. Avoid shaking or fluffing linen:
a. to avoid causing a draft
b. to prevent germs from spreading
c. to avoid dropping the linen
d. to avoid making noise

26. The only way to find out if you have HBV is:
a. blood test
b. vaccine
c. x-ray
d. urine test

27. People infected with HIV:
a. show symptoms of the disease within a few days
b. are carriers for life
c. always know they are infected
d. will recover in six months to a year

28. For perineal care, always wipe:
a. from front to back
b. from back to front
c. in whichever direction is easiest
d. back and forth two times

29. For a tub bath, the best water temperature is generally:
   a. 80 degrees F
   b. 90 degrees F
   c. 105 degrees F
   d. 115 degrees F

30. After you have tested the water temperature:
   a. help the resident out of the tub
   b. have the resident check the water temperature
   c. leave the room
   d. open the window for ventilation

31. Foot care is given only by licensed staff if the resident:
   a. takes any medications
   b. has poor circulation or is diabetic
   c. wants special treatment
   d. is aggressive

32. If a resident is unconscious, mouth care should be given:
   a. once a day
   b. at least twice a day
   c. every two hours
   d. only as necessary

33. Areas of the body at high risk of pressure ulcers are:
   a. fatty tissues
   b. bony areas
   c. nose and throat
   d. upper arms

34. Help prevent dehydration by:
   a. cutting back on fluid intake
   b. encouraging fluid intake
   c. bathing twice a day
   d. withholding fluids

35. People who are incontinent:
   a. should be scolded when they have an "accident"
   b. are usually too lazy to go to the bathroom
   c. sometimes regain bladder control with appropriate training
   d. should restrict their fluid intake

36. A catheter is:
   a. a tube inserted into the bladder
   b. an opening created by surgery
   c. a feeding tube
   d. a suppository

37. A thermometer measures:
   a. respiration
   b. blood pressure
   c. body temperature
   d. systolic pressure

38. To take the temperature of a resident who is wearing an oxygen mask, you would:
   a. remove the mask to take an oral reading
   b. chart that the temperature was not taken
   c. take a rectal, aural, or axillary temperature
   d. feel the resident's forehead

39. Taking a pulse measures:
   a. respiration
   b. blood pressure
   c. activity
   d. heartbeat

40. The radial pulse is located in the:
   a. neck
   b. wrist
   c. temple
   d. foot

41. One respiration equals:
a. one inspiration and one expiration
b. two full breaths
c. two inspirations
d. one inhalation

42. Hypertension is:
a. low blood pressure
b. lack of blood pressure
c. high pulse rate
d. high blood pressure

43. Good nutrition is based on:
a. eating a variety of foods every day
b. counting calories
c. measuring fluid intake and output
d. exercising

44. Serving the wrong meal to a person:
a. is never a problem
b. is okay, but be more careful next time
c. makes more work for yourself
d. can cause severe problems

45. The best way to prevent accidents is:
a. telling residents to be careful
b. getting angry when a resident has an accident
c. placing the call signal out of a resident's reach
d. being alert to safety hazards

46. The LEADING cause of injury to the elderly is:
a. falling
b. burns
c. accidental poisoning
d. choking

47. Cleansers and disinfectants should be:
a. readily available
b. kept in open cupboards
c. locked in storage areas
d. kept in handy locations

48. The universal sign for choking is:
a. coughing
b. clutching the stomach
c. clutching the throat
d. dysphagia

49. The abdominal thrust procedure is used only when:
a. there is a complete obstruction of the airway
b. a person is comatose
c. a person complains of chest pains
d. a person asks for help

50. CPR means:
a. cardiopulmonary restrictions
b. cerebral pulmonary resuscitation
c. cardiopulmonary resuscitation
d. cardiopulmonary post resuscitation

51. Restraints are used only when:
a. the staff is busy
b. a doctor orders the restraints
c. the resident is behaving badly
d. you think it is necessary for the resident's safety

52. Reality orientation is used:
a. for people who cannot remember recent events
b. to help people remember past events
c. to introduce residents to the facility
d. to introduce new staff to the facility

53. The FIRST thing you should do if a person has a seizure is:
a. leave the room to find help
b. hold the person's hand
c. restrain the person
d. protect the person from injury

54. The medical term for a stroke is:
a. cardiovascular accident
b. cerebrovascular accident
c. brain damage
d. myocardial infarction

55. It is important for you to:
a. encourage the residents to be independent
b. dress and feed the residents, even when they are able to dress and feed themselves
c. discourage the residents from talking about their problems
d. tell the family about the resident's problems

56. If people are able to assist with their personal care, you would:
a. provide the care yourself because it is faster and easier
b. tell them to hurry
c. let people do it, even if it takes more time and effort than doing it yourself
d. discourage people from trying

57. ROM is important because the exercises:
a. give the resident something to do
b. keep you busy
c. maintain mobility and prevent atrophy
d. cause contractures

58. Long periods of immobility cause:
a. elevated pulse rate
b. dysphagia
c. myocardial infarction
d. contractures and atrophy

59. If something seems wrong with a resident, you would:
a. check on the person in an hour
b. do nothing until you know what the problem is
c. report it
d. tell the person's family

60. During the final stages of life, you would:
a. leave the person alone
b. continue normal care
c. discourage visitors
d. keep the room dark

True/False

61. T F Nursing Assistants have a legal and moral responsibility to keep information about the residents confidential.

62. T F Good listening skills are important for Nursing Assistants.

63. T F HIV/AIDS cannot be prevented.

64. T F Never wear gloves when handling blood or body fluids.

65. **T F** Washing your hands is the most important preventive measure for infection control.

66. **T F** Hypotension is high blood pressure.

67. **T F** Fluid measurements are recorded in cubic centimeters.

68. **T F** Incontinence is bowel elimination that is infrequent and painful.

69. **T F** Proper body mechanics help prevent back injuries.

70. **T F** Aging skin is fragile and damages easily.

71. **T F** Your attitude and behavior do not affect the resident's behavior.

72. **T F** In case of fire, the FIRST step is to locate a fire extinguisher.

73. **T F** The FIRST sign that a pressure ulcer is developing is a break in the skin.

74. **T F** All complaints from residents about the facility should be reported.

75. **T F** Nursing Assistants should allow residents to make personal choices whenever possible.

Correct Answers

					75. T	74. T	73. F	72. F	71. F
70. T	69. T	68. F	67. T	66. F	65. T	64. F	63. F	62. T	61. T
60. b	59. c	58. d	57. c	56. c	55. a	54. b	53. d	52. a	51. b
50. c	49. a	48. c	47. c	46. a	45. d	44. d	43. a	42. d	41. a
40. b	39. d	38. c	37. c	36. a	35. c	34. b	33. b	32. c	31. b
30. b	29. c	28. a	27. b	26. a	25. b	24. a	23. a	22. a	21. d
20. c	19. d	18. b	17. a	16. d	15. b	14. a	13. b	12. c	11. b
10. a	9. d	8. a	7. c	6. a	5. b	4. d	3. b	2. d	1. c

155

Continuing Your Education

Take advantage of every opportunity to upgrade your skills.

Continuing education is vital for *everyone* in the healthcare profession. Stay on top of trends and research, and make the most of your career. Take advantage of every opportunity to upgrade your skills. Be the best Nursing Assistant you can be. Benefits include a rewarding career and personal satisfaction.

- Stay current with CPR and first aid training.
- Attend classes and workshops.
- Be enthusiastic about in-service training.
- Ask questions (and remember the answers).
- Practice and improve your skills.

- Learn from mistakes.
- Read, research, and be curious about new information
- Search the internet; there is an amazing wealth of information to be found!

Resources Available from First Class Books

The ***Instructor's Guide*** is a valuable resource for new and experienced trainers. It is jam-packed with hundreds of creative training tips and ideas, hands-on activities, practice tests, and more. Designed as a companion for *Nursing Assistant, A Basic Study Guide*, the Instructor's Guide is compatible with *any* training program. It comes in a handy three-ring binder.

The ***Student Workbook*** provides learning activities and practice tests to prepare students for successful completion of the certification exam.

Pocket-size booklets:

Dementia, Providing Gentle Care focuses on quality care for victims of dementia (including Alzheimer's disease). Sections include recognizing symptoms, understanding dementia, communicating effectively, managing difficult behavior and supporting family and friends.

Test Tips for the Nursing Assistant Certification Exam offers test-taking tips and a variety of practice exams.

Cultural Awareness, Building Positive Relationships is a "must" for today's multi-cultural workplace. Topics include culture shock, cultural awareness, communication, health issues, and more.

Growing Old, Handle with Care, helps caregivers recognize normal signs of aging, alerts them to common health problems of the elderly, and provides details for quality care.

Medical Abbreviations

Healthcare workers need to be familiar with medical abbreviations.

$\bar{a}$	before		FF	force fluids
abd	abdomen		fld (fl)	fluid
a.c.	before meals		ft	foot or feet
AD	Alzheimer's disease		Fx	fracture
ADLs	activities of daily living		gal	gallon
AED	automated electronic defibrillator		GI	gastrointestinal
Adm (adm)	admission		GU	genitourinary
ad lib	as desired		h (hr)	hour
AM (am)	morning (before noon)		H_2O	water
amb	ambulate		HOB	head of bed
amt	amount		HOH	hard of hearing
AROM	active range of motion		h.s.	bedtime (hour of sleep)
ax	axillary (armpit)		ht	height
b.i.d.	twice a day		Hx	history
BM (bm)	bowel movement		ICU	Intensive Care Unit
BP	blood pressure		in	inch
BRP	bathroom privileges		I&O	intake and output
C	Celsius or Centigrade		IV	intravenous
$\bar{c}$	with		L	liter
CA	cancer		lb	pound
Cath	catheter		liq	liquid
CBC	complete blood count		LE	lower extremity
CBR	complete bed rest		LLE	left lower extremity
cc	cubic centimeter		LPN	licensed practical nurse
CCU	coronary care unit		L (lt)	left
CHD	coronary heart disease		LUE	left upper extremity
CHF	congestive heart failure		LLQ	left lower quadrant of abdomen
CN	charge nurse		LUQ	left upper quadrant of abdomen
C/O	complains of		LVN	licensed vocational nurse
COPD	chronic obstructive pulmonary disease		meds	medications
CPR	cardiopulmonary resuscitation		mid noc	midnight
CVA	cerebrovascular accident (stroke)		min	minute
DC (d/c)	discontinue		MI	myocardial infarction
DON	director of nursing		mL	milliliter
DOA	dead on arrival		mm	millimeters
DNR	do not resuscitate		neg	negative
Dr.	doctor		nl	normal
Drsg	dressing		no	number
Dx	diagnosis		noc	night
ECG	(EKG) electrocardiogram		NPO	nothing by mouth
EEG	electroencephalogram		N/V	nausea and vomiting
ER	emergency room		O_2	oxygen
ENT	ear, nose, throat		OD	right eye
F	Fahrenheit		OU	both eyes
FBS	fasting blood sugar		OS	left eye

oob	out of bed	s̄	without
OT	occupational therapist	Sx	symptoms
oz	ounce	spec	specimen
p̄	after	SOB	shortness of breath
pc	after meals	staph	staphylococcus (bacteria)
po	by mouth (oral)	STAT	immediately
PM (p.m.)	after noon	strep	streptococcus (bacteria)
p.r.n.	as needed	tab	tablet
PROM	passive range of motion	tbsp	tablespoon
pt	patient/resident	TIA	transient ischemmic attack
PT	physical therapy	t.i.d.	three times a day
q.d.	every day	TPR	temperature, pulse, respiration
q.i.d.	four times a day	tsp	teaspoon
q.h.	every hour	Tx	treatment
q.o.d.	every other day	U/A	urinalysis
R	rectal	UE	upper extremity
RN	registered nurse	UP	Universal Precautions
ROM	range of motion	URI	upper respiratory infection
R (rt)	right	UTI	urinary tract infection
RLE	right lower extremity	VS	vital signs
RUE	right upper extremity	WBC	white blood cell count
RLQ	right lower quadrant of abdomen	W/C	wheelchair
RUQ	right upper quadrant of abdomen	wt	weight
Rx	prescription		

Practical Use of Abbreviations

Abbreviations are important for understanding instructions in healthcare facilities. Avoid using abbreviations when you are communicating with the residents, families, or the public.

Examples

1. amb c̄ walker b.i.d.
ambulate with walker two times a day

2. dresses s̄ supervision
dresses without supervision

3. elevate HOB p.r.n. SOB
raise head of bed as needed for shortness of breath

4. assist c̄ ROM t.i.d.
assist with range of motion three times a day

5. give 1 tab t.i.d. a.c.
give one tablet three times a day before meals

Practice

1. Pt c/o headache

_____

2. Report to CN STAT

_____

3. TPR b.i.d.

_____

4. Amb q.i.d.

_____

5. Reposition pt q.h.

_____

Glossary of Terms

Learn to recognize common terms used in healthcare.

The brief definitions used in this glossary are a quick reference based on how the words are used within the context of this book. For complete and "official" definitions, refer to a dictionary.

A

ADLs	activities of daily living, everyday tasks that involve personal care
AED	automated external defibrillator, portable device used to restore regular heart rhythm
AIDS	Acquired Immune Deficiency Syndrome, disease that attacks the immune system, preventing the body from fighting infection
abdominal thrusts	series of rapid thrusts to the abdomen in an effort to clear the airway
abduction	moving body part away from normal position
abuse	physical, mental, or sexual harm, exploitation, or neglect
acceptance	resigning oneself to circumstances
acetest	test to detect acetone
acidosis	inability of blood to get rid of toxins
adduction	moving body part toward the body
advocate	spokesperson or representative
agonal respiration	inadequate labored breathing or gasping
airway	passage for air to the lungs
alignment	keeping a straight line
Alzheimer's disease	a progressive, incurable brain disease that affects memory, judgment, and personality

a.m.	morning hours beginning at midnight and ending at noon
ambulate	walk
anatomy	body structure
anal, anus	rectum
apical pulse	pulse felt at the apex of the heart, under the left breast
aphasia	difficulty using or understanding words
arteries	blood vessels that carry blood away from the heart to the system
arteriosclerosis	thickening and hardening of the arterial walls
asepsis	procedures to reduce pathogens
aspiration	breathing solids or fluids into the lungs
assault	an unlawful personal attack
assistive devices	aids to help people regain lost functions
atherosclerosis	blockage of the arteries by fatty substances
atrial fibrillation	(AF) irregular rate or rhythm of heartbeat
atrophy	wasting away of muscle or tissue
aural	relating to the ear
autoclave	intense heat sterilization
axilla/axillary	armpit

B

BP cuff	instrument for measuring blood pressure
bacteria	disease-causing germs
bargaining	making a deal
barrier	obstacle blocking approach, path, or goal
basic needs	physical, emotional, mental, and social requirements
battery	an attack when an actual blow is delivered
bedpan	a pan used for elimination while confined to bed
beliefs	individual viewpoints, feelings, and opinions
bladder	organ that holds urine before it is excreted
blood pressure	force of blood against walls of blood vessels
body mechanics	proper body positioning
body systems	interdependent systems that make up the structure and function of the body
brachial pulse	pulse point at the inside elbow

C

CDC	Center for Disease Control, a governmental agency
CHD	coronary heart disease
COPD	chronic obstructive pulmonary disease
CPR	cardiopulmonary resuscitation, first aid procedure for sudden cardiac or respiratory arrest
CVA	cerebrovascular accident, stroke
cancer	a malignant tumor that grows, spreads, and destroys

care plan	detailed care instructions for each resident
cardiovascular	pertaining to heart and blood vessels
carotid pulse	pulse point on each side of the neck
cataract	clouding of the lens of the eye
catheter	drain tube for bladder
centimeter	metric measure equal to 1/100 meter or .3937 inch
cerebral	pertaining to the brain
chart	medical record of health and care
certification	license to work
chemotherapy	treatment using drugs
choking	response to an obstruction in the airway
clinical skills	hands-on procedures
clinitest	urine test for sugar
coccyx	tailbone
cognitively impaired	difficulty in processing information
combustible	any material that will ignite and burn easily
commode	movable chair containing a built-in bedpan
communication	exchanging information (talking, writing, gestures, etc.)
compassion	sympathy for another's suffering
concise	to the point
confidentiality	not revealing personal information about others
confusion	mentally unclear or uncertain
constipation	difficult or painful bowel movement

contaminate	to infect by contact with a non-sterile object
contracture	shortening and tightening of muscle or joint
contra-indicated	not advisable
crutch	support that fits under the armpit
custom	long-established practice or belief
CVA	cerebrovascular accident, stroke
cyanosis	bluish color of skin due to lack of oxygen
cystitis	bladder infection

D

decubitus ulcer	pressure sore
defamation	oral or written words that damage someone's reputation
defecate	eliminating waste from the bowel
defense mechanisms	a self-protective response to a real or imagined threat
defibrillate	to apply an electric shock to the chest or heart
deformity	badly formed body structure
degenerate	decline from a former or normal condition
dehydration	too little fluid in body tissues
dementia	loss or impairment of mental powers
denial	refusing to believe
dentures	false teeth
depression	low spirits, sadness, dejection
dermis	inner layer of skin
diabetes	chronic disease, pancreas does not secrete enough insulin
diastolic pressure	lowest pressure, when the heart is relaxed

diet card	order card indicating special diet or restrictions
dietician	health professional specializing in meal planning and preparation
digestion	process of dissolving and breaking down food
disinfection	killing or slowing the growth of most microorganisms
document	official written report that supports observations
drawsheet	sheet used to move a person in bed
dry dressing	material used to cover a wound
dysphagia	swallowing difficulty

E

edema	swelling, excess collection of fluids in tissue
elasticity	flexibility
elder abuse	the mistreatment of an elderly person
elimination	the process of removing wastes from the body
embolus	blood clot or abnormal particle circulated in the blood (e.g., air bubble)
emesis	vomit
empathy	sharing another's emotions
emotional and social needs	basic requirements for contentment and companionship
enema	injecting fluids into the rectum
epidermis	outer layer of skin
epiglottis	covers the opening of the windpipe during swallowing
epilepsy	chronic disease of the nervous system characterized by seizures
erection	in males, when the penis becomes rigid

ethics	a standard of conduct
excrete	pass, discharge
expiration	breathing out
extremity	limb of the body (arm, leg)

F

false documentation	knowingly recording incorrect information on a resident's record
feces	body waste from the bowel, stool
feedback	method to determine whether a message is understood
feeding tubes	special tubes passed into the stomach for providing nourishment
femoral pulse	pulse point in the groin (where abdomen joins thigh)
fiber	roughage essential for proper elimination
first aid	emergency care until medical help arrives
flaccid	weak and limp
flow sheet	record of daily care and activities
fluid balance	maintaining the right amount of body fluids
friction	rubbing one surface against another

G

GI	gastro (stomach) intestinal, digestive system
gait	stride or walk
gait belt	wide belt used to assist with ambulating (also called transfer belt)
gastronomy	opening made to stomach for feeding
gesture	body movements that express an idea
glaucoma	increased pressure in the eye

glucose	sugar
grand mal seizure	convulsions resulting in loss of consciousness
grief	reaction to loss
grievance	formal complaint

H

HBV	Hepatitis B Virus, viral infection of the liver
HIV	Human Immunodeficiency Virus which causes AIDS
healthcare team	everyone who provides care for a person
hearing impaired	loss of hearing, deafness
heart disease	abnormal conditions including vessels, rhythms, infection, defects
Heimlich Maneuver	see abdominal thrust procedure
hemiplegia	paralysis on one side of the body
hemiparesis	muscular weakness on one side of the body
hemorrhage	bleeding
HIPAA	health information privacy, governmental rules and regulations
home health agency	organization that employs and places home health aides
homeostasis	in balance
hygiene	principles of being clean and sanitary
hyperglycemia	abnormally high levels of sugar in the blood
hypertension	blood pressure higher than normal
hypoglycemia	abnormally low level of sugar in the blood
hypotension	blood pressure lower than normal

I

immobile	unable to move
immune	not subject to a particular disease because of the presence of antibodies
immune system	body defense mechanism to protect against disease
impaction	inability to pass feces
incontinence	inability to control bladder and/or bowel functions
independence	self-managing, not relying on others
individuality	unique qualities that set each person apart from others
infection	invasion of disease-producing microorganisms
infection prevention/control	methods used to stop the spread of disease
inflammation	tissue redness, pain, swelling
insomnia	inability to commence or maintain sleep
inspiration	breathing in
insulin	hormone produced by the pancreas which breaks down sugar and starches
insulin shock	condition resulting from too much insulin or too little food
intake/output	measure of fluid taken in and voided
integumentary system	outer covering of skin, also hair and nails
intervention	action taken in order to prevent something
intravenous	going directly into the vein
isolation	separating from others

K

kilogram	metric measure of weight equal to 2.2046 pounds

L

labia	folds of skin at entrance to vagina
legal action	steps to enforce the law or to punish violators
lethargy	abnormal drowsiness or lack of energy
life-threatening	emergency condition that could end in death
lift sheet	sheet used to move a resident
linen	bedding, towels, gowns, masks, and other articles that require disinfection or disposal
liter	metric measure of volume, equal to 33.8 fluid ounces or 1.056 liquid quart or .908 dry quart
log rolling	method for moving a person onto his or her side (by rolling like a log)

M

mandatory reporting	required reporting of susptected abuse or neglect
Maslow, Abraham	psychologist whose theory of the hierarchy of human needs helps explain behavior
measurement	dimensions, capacity, or amount
medical asepsis	procedure to reduce pathogens
metabolism	process by which energy is made available for use by the body
meter	metric measure of length, equal to 39.37 inches
metric system	decimal system of weights and measures
microorganism	living organism seen only with a microscope

milliliter	one thousandth of a liter
mitered corners	corners of a bed sheet forming a triangle and tucked under the mattress
mobility	ability to move
mobility aids	devices to help residents walk and move more easily
monkey pole	bar above the bed to help a person move or exercise
move	to change place or position
myocardial infarction	(MI) heart attack

N

NPO	nothing by mouth, no food or beverages consumed by mouth
nasogastric tube (Ng tube)	soft plastic tube inserted through nose into stomach for feeding and/or medicating
negligence	failure to provide necessary care
non-ambulatory	cannot walk
nonverbal	non-spoken expression, body language, facial expressions, hand gestures, etc.
nutrients	substances in food that are necessary for life
nutrition	food science related to health, process of nourishing the body

O

objective reporting	facts only
observe	watch, pay close attention
obstruction	blockage
oral hygiene	care of the teeth, mouth, and gums

organism	living matter
OSHA	Occupational Safety & Health Administration, a governmental agency
osteoporosis	bones become brittle and fracture easily

P

pacemaker	device that regulates heartbeat
paralysis	loss of voluntary movement
paraphrase	repeat statement in your own words
pathogen	disease-causing microorganism
pedal pulse	pulse site at top of foot
perineal care	cleansing of the rectal and genital areas
personal hygiene	cleanliness and grooming
personal protective equipment	(PPE) gloves, gowns, masks, safety glasses, face shields, etc.
petit mal	a partial seizure which does not result in loss of consciousness
physiology	how the body functions
p.m.	evening hours beginning at 12 noon and ending at midnight
pneumonia	infection of the lungs
podiatrist	foot doctor
policy	regulation, definite plan of what is to be done
popliteal pulse	pulse point at back of knee
positioning	how a person is placed, sitting, lying, or standing
postmortem	after death
practical skills	hands-on training, practice, and performance
precautions	measures taken beforehand against possible danger

preference	choice, like better or best
pressure ulcers	body sores caused by pressure, also called decubitus ulcers
procedure	steps to follow in a particular order
prone	lying on the stomach
prosthesis	artificial body part
protect	defend, keep safe
protective barriers	coverings to guard against infection (gloves, masks, gowns, safety glasses, face shields, etc.)
protective devices	equipment used to protect and support the residents, restraints
psychomotor seizures	temporary loss of judgment and motor control
pulse	throbbing of the arteries caused by contractions of the heart
pulse oximeter	blood oxygen monitoring device

R

ROM	range of motion, movement of joint through its normal range of activity
radial pulse	heartbeat felt at the wrist
radiation	therapy using high-energy waves
reality orientation	maintaining awareness of person, place, and time
recovery position	specific positioning used after an accident to prevent choking and to protect breathing
rehabilitation	restoring a person's physical and/or mental abilities
reliability	dependability, accountability
reminisce	recall past experiences
report	giving detailed information
reprisal	revenge on another person
requirements	necessary knowledge or skills

rescue breathing	artificial respirations used in CPR
resigned	to give up deliberately
resources	available services and information
respect/dignity	high regard for another person
respiration	breathing, consisting of one inspiration and one expiration
responsibility	being accountable
restorative	bring back what was lost
restraint	protective device that restricts or limits movement
rights	standards of justice, law, and morality
role	expectations and limits
rotation	circlular
rupture	the tearing apart of tissue

S

safety hazard	dangerous condition, obstacle to security
seizure	disorder that may include convulsions
self-actualization	self-esteem, personal pride
self-esteem	personal pride, feeling good about oneself
self-managing	capable of caring for oneself
sensory	pertaining to the senses (seeing, hearing, touching, smelling, etc.)
sensitivity	showing concern for another's feelings
sexuality	characteristics or feelings pertaining to sex
shock	severe reaction to an event that can cause the cardiovascular system to shut down
significant others	everyone who is important to a person

skin care	cleansing and protection of the skin	transfer	move from one place to another
slander	spoken statement that damages another's reputation	transient ischemic attack	(TIA) mini-stroke, usually lasting only a few minutes and causing no permanent damage
slide board	board used to transfer people if there is no danger of spinal injury	transmit	to pass from one object or person to another
spasm	involuntary muscle contraction	transfer belt	a wide belt worn around the waist to provide a grip for lifting or supporting a person (same as gait belt)
specimen	sample of body material		
sphygmoma-nometer	instrument to measure blood pressure		
sputum	mucus expelled from the lungs		
stance	the way a person stands, with special attention to placement of feet	**U**	
Standard Precautions	safety measures used for all body fluids and air-borne pathogens	Universal Precautions	safety measures used with blood and body fluids
sterile	absence of all disease-producing microorganisms	urinal	container used by males for urinating
stethoscope	instrument used to hear sounds in the body	urine	liquid waste from the kidneys
stool	feces, body waste from the bowels	**V**	
stroke	rupture, blockage, or clotting of a blood vessel in the brain	vein	blood vessel that carries blood to the heart
subjective	includes feelings and impressions	verbal	spoken words
susceptible	easily affected by	vertebrae	bones of the spinal column
supine	lying on the back	vital signs	temperature, respiration, pulse, and blood pressure
systolic pressure	highest pressure, when the heart contracts	visually impaired	blindness or loss of sight
		void	empty bowels or bladder
T		**W**	
therapeutic	beneficial treatment	walker	tubular frame used as a support for walking
thermometer	instrument for measuring temperature	wellness	absence of illness
thrombus	blood clot	wheelchair	chair mounted on wheels
timely	promptly, at the right time		

Index

POCKET REFERENCE—Abbreviations 2

Activities   Elimination

Activities	Elimination
ADLs	BM
amb	BRP
W/C	UA
ROM	spec
PT	I&O

POCKET REFERENCE—Abbreviations 4

Instructions

PO	c̄
NPO	s̄
H₂O	SBA
DC or d/c	DNR

POCKET REFERENCE—Abbreviations 1

Amounts

amt	cc
tbsp	L
tsp	mL
oz	nil
gal	qt

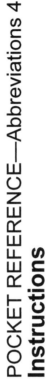

POCKET REFERENCE—Abbreviations 3

Measurements

ht	F
wt	C
ft	kg
in	lb

Tips and Terms Flash Cards

Activities

activities of daily living

ambulate

wheelchair

range of motion

physical therapy

Elimination

bowel movement

bathroom privileges

urinalysis

specimen

intake and output

Amounts

amount

tablespoon

teaspoon

ounce

gallon

liter

milliliter

cubic centimeter

quart

Instructions

by mouth (oral)

nothing by mouth

water

discontinue

with

without

stand-by assistance
(ready to assist as needed)

do not resuscitate

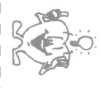

Measurements

height

weight

feet

inches

Fahrenheit

Centigrade

kilogram

pound

POCKET REFERENCE—Abbreviations 5
Body Parts

pt	GI
abd	GU
R	ENT
ax	L or lt
aural	R or rt

POCKET REFERENCE—Abbreviations 6
Body Parts

RLQ	LLE
LLQ	LUE
RUQ	RLE
LUQ	RUE

POCKET REFERENCE   Abbreviations 7
Abbreviations   Diagnostics

Rx	Dx
IV	EEG
O₂	EKG or ECG
FF	RBC
CBR	WBC

POCKET REFERENCE—Abbreviations 8
Specific Disorders

MI	COPD
CHF	CHD
CVA	TIA
CA	AD
UTI	URI

Tips and Terms Flash Cards

Body Parts

right lower quadrant	left lower extremity
left lower quadrant	left upper extremity
right upper quadrant	right lower extremity
left upper quadrant	right upper extremity

Body Parts

patient	gastrointestinal (stomach and intestine)
abdomen	genitourinary (genital and urinary organs)
rectal	ears, nose, throat
axillary (armpit)	left
relating to the ear	right

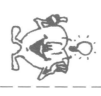

Specific Disorders

myocardial infarction (heart attack)	chronic obstructive pulmonary disease
congestive heart failure	coronary heart disease
cerebral vascular accident (stroke)	transient ischemic attack
cancer	Alzheimer's disease
urinary tract infection	upper respiratory infection

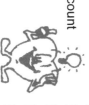
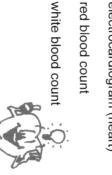

Abbreviations   Diagnostics

prescription	diagnosis
intravenous	electroencephalogram (brain waves)
oxygen	electrocardiogram (heart)
force fluids	red blood count
complete bed rest	white blood count

POCKET REFERENCE—Abbreviations 9
Time (when)   Time (frequency)

ā
p̄
a.c.
p.c.
ad lib
p.r.n.
STAT

q.h.
q.d.
q.o.d.
b.i.d.
t.i.d.
q.i.d.

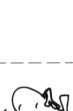

POCKET REFERENCE—Abbreviations 10
Time of Day

AM or a.m.   Noon

PM or p.m.   Midnight

noc   Military time

h.s.

POCKET REFERENCE—Abbreviations 11
Vital Signs

VS   sphygmomanometer

TPR   stethoscope

BP

POCKET REFERENCE—Abbreviations 12
Complications

SOB

HOH

c/o

Fx

staph

Tips and Terms Flash Cards

Time of Day

morning

afternoon or evening

night

bedtime (hour of sleep)

12:00 PM

12:00 AM

based on 24 hr clock

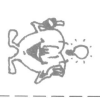

Time (when)

before

after

before meals

after meals

as desired

as necessary

immediately

every hour

every day

every other day

two times a day

three times a day

four times a day

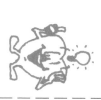

Complications

shortness of breath

hard of hearing

complains of

fracture

staphylococcus (bacteria)

Vital Signs

vital signs

temperature, pulse, respiration

blood pressure

device used to take BP

device used to listen to heart and lungs

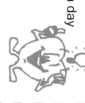

POCKET REFERENCE—Observations 1
Pneumonia

Describe:

List symptoms:

Action to take:

POCKET REFERENCE—Observations 3
Alzheimer's Disease/Dementia

Describe:

List symptoms:

Action to take:

POCKET REFERENCE—Word Parts 1
Medical Conditions

-emia   -oma

-uria   -plegia

-itis   -phasia

-stomy   -rrhage

-stasis   -rrhea

-pathy

POCKET REFERENCE—Observations 2
Diabetes Complications

List complications:

List symptoms for each:

Action to take:

Tips and Terms Flash Cards

Pneumonia

Description: acute lung disease

Symptoms:
coughing
pain in chest
feverish
congested

Action: report and chart

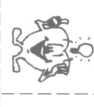

Medical Conditions

blood condition — tumor

urine condition — paralysis

inflammation — speaking

creation of an opening — excessive flow

maintaining — flow or discharge

disease

Alzheimer's Disease/Dementia

Description: progressive mental deterioration

Symptoms:
unable to remember recent events
increased confusion
decreased attention span
tires easily
uncontrolled behavior
increased anxiety

Action:
report and chart changes in behavior; be patient; give simple instructions, one step at a time; supervise closely

Diabetes Complications

Diabetic coma symptoms:
comes on gradually
acetone breath (smells fruity)
increased urination
thirsty
nausea
heavy breathing
flushed, hot, dry skin
high blood sugar

Insulin shock symptoms:
comes on suddenly
weak, dizzy, trembling
perspiring
vision problems
hungry
shallow respiration
pale, cold, clammy
low blood sugar

Action: life-threatening; report immediately

POCKET REFERENCE—Observations 4
Cardiac Arrest

Describe:

List symptoms:

Action to take:

POCKET REFERENCE—Observations 5
Choking

Describe:

List symptoms:

Action to take:

POCKET REFERENCE—Observations 6
Cerebrovascular Accident (CVA)

Describe:

List symptoms:

Action to take:

POCKET REFERENCE—Observations 7
Depression

Describe:

List symptoms:

Action to take:

Tips and Terms Flash Cards

Choking

Description: completely obstructed airway

Symptoms: clutching the throat
unable to breathe
cannot speak or cough

Action: life-threatening; call for help
immediately; begin the abdominal
thrust procedure

Cardiac Arrest

Description: sudden, abrupt loss of heart function

Symptoms: sudden collapse (without warning)
loss of consciousness
no breathing
no pulse

Action: life-threatening; call for help
immediately; begin CPR

Depression

Description: acute sadness

Symptoms: loss of appetite
withdrawn
low self-esteem
lack of interest or enthusiasm

Action: report and chart changes; express
concern and interest; take time
to talk (but don't force conversation); motivate to participate
in activities; help to feel good
about self and appearance

Cerebrovascular Accident (CVA)

Description: caused by blood clot, build up of plaque,
or bleeding in the brain

Symptoms: paralysis on one side
loss of sensation on one side
eyelid or mouth droops
spasms or loss of muscle control
speech problems

Action: report and chart changes in
condition; supervise carefully to
protect from injury; encourage
and praise independence

POCKET REFERENCE—Observations 8
Urinary Tract Infection (UTI)

Describe:

List symptoms:

List some causes:

Action to take:

POCKET REFERENCE—Observations 9
Allergic Reaction

Describe:

List symptoms:

Action to take:

POCKET REFERENCE—Observations 10
Myocardial Infarction (MI)

Describe:

List symptoms:

Action to take:

POCKET REFERENCE—Observations 11
Congestive Heart Failure (CHF)

Describe:

List symptoms:

Action to take:

Tips and Terms Flash Cards

Allergic Reaction

Description: hypersensitivity to certain things

Symptoms:
itching or tingling
skin rashes
rapid swelling
breathing difficulty
vision problems
scratchy throat

Action:
emergency situation;
report immediately

Urinary Tract Infection (UTI)

Description: infection of the urinary system

Symptoms:
pain in lower back
pain or burning with urination
change in urine odor, color, frequency

Some causes:
insufficient fluids
poor perineal care
unable to empty bladder completely
indwelling catheter
bedridden/inactivity

Action:
report and chart; encourage fluids

Congestive Heart Failure (CHF)

Description: circulatory congestion

Symptoms:
lung congestion
chest discomfort
swelling in extremities
weight gain
restlessness
breathing difficulty
dizzy, confused, tired

Action:
emergency situation;
get help immediately

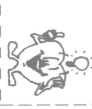

Myocardial Infarction (MI)

Description: heart attack

Symptoms:
chest pain
pale, cold, clammy
pain in left arm and neck
irregular, weak pulse
decreased blood pressure

Action:
life-threatening;
report immediately

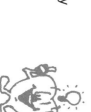

POCKET REFERENCE—Observations 13
Dehydration

Describe:

List symptoms:

Action to take:

POCKET REFERENCE—Observations 15
Pressure Ulcer

Describe:

Cause:

List symptoms:

Action to take:

POCKET REFERENCE—Observations 12
Edema

Describe:

List symptoms:

Action to take:

POCKET REFERENCE—Observations 14
Approaching Death

Describe:

List symptoms:

Action to take:

Cut along dashed lines for pocket size reference cards.

Tips and Terms Flash Cards

Dehydration

Description: lack of fluids; affects all body systems

Symptoms:
excessive thirst
decreased urine output
constipation
dry skin, lips, tongue
decreased blood pressure
rapid, weak pulse

Action:
can be life-threatening;
report immediately

Edema

Description: fluid retention

Symptoms:
swelling (feet, ankles, face, fingers, joints, tissues)
weight gain
decreased urine output

Action:
report and chart changes;
elevate swollen area;
encourage loose-fitting clothing

Pressure Ulcer

Description: decubitus ulcer, bed/pressure sore

Cause: pressure on body parts that are not protected by fatty tissues.

Symptoms:
redness that does not disappear when pressure is relieved
area is tender and warmer than other skin
blisters or open sores that can lead to infection

Action:
keep skin clean and dry; massage gently;
keep bed free of wrinkles; encourage
fluids; reposition frequently; cushion and
bridge body parts as needed; report and
chart

Approaching Death

Description: final stages of life

Symptoms:
cold hands and feet
blank stare
pale or gray
perspiring
limp
slow or difficult breathing
rattling sound in throat or chest
rapid, weak pulse

Action:
report immediately; continue giving the
best care possible; keep the room well
ventilated and lighted; offer comfort
and support to the patient and the
family; provide privacy with loved ones

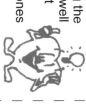

Cut along dashed lines for pocket size reference cards.

Temperature Conversion

°C ↔ °F		°C ↔ °F		°C ↔ °F	
35.0	95.0	38.0	100.4	39.4	102.9
36.0	96.8	38.2	100.8	39.6	103.3
37.0	**98.6**	38.4	101.2	39.8	103.7
37.2	99.0	38.6	101.5	40.0	104.0
37.4	99.3	38.8	101.8	40.2	104.3
37.6	99.7	39.0	102.2	40.4	104.7
37.8	100.1	39.2	102.6	40.6	105.1

Time Conversion Chart

24 Hour	12 Hour	24 Hour	12 Hour
0000 MIDNIGHT	12 AM	1200 NOON	12 PM
0100	1 AM	1300	1 PM
0200	2 AM	1400	2 PM
0300	3 AM	1500	3 PM
0400	4 AM	1600	4 PM
0500	5 AM	1700	5 PM
0600	6 AM	1800	6 PM
0700	7 AM	1900	7 PM
0800	8 AM	2000	8 PM
0900	9 AM	2100	9 PM
1000	10 AM	2200	10 PM
1100	11 AM	2300	11 PM

My Emergency Information

9-1-1 or

- Fire _____
- Medical _____
- Police _____
- Poison Control _____

Facility _____

Physical Address _____

Contact Person _____

Contact Phone _____

Pain Assessment Tool

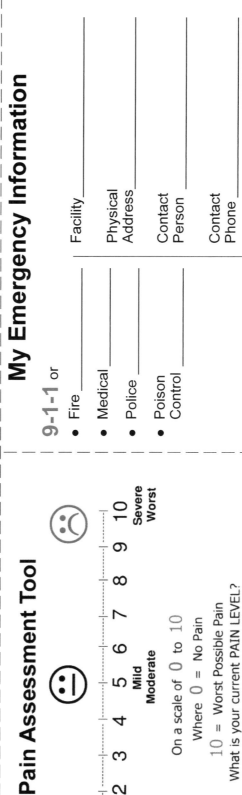

0 1 2 3 4 5 6 7 8 9 10

0 No Pain

5 Mild Moderate

10 Severe Worst

On a scale of 0 to 10

Where 0 = No Pain

10 = Worst Possible Pain

What is your current PAIN LEVEL?

Reference Tools Reference Card

183

Formula for Temperature Conversion

To convert Fahrenheit temperature into Celcius:
1. Begin by subtracting 32 from the Fahrenheit number.
2. Divide the answer by 9.
3. Then multiply that answer by 5.

To convert Celcius temperature into Fahrenheit:
1. Begin by multiplying the Celcius temperature by 9,
2. Divide the answer by 5.
3. Now add 32.

Time Conversion

- **AM** - Midnight to Noon
- **PM** - Noon to Midnight

- **Military Time** - based on a **24-hour** clock

Military time begins at Midnight with Zero Hour

Following are examples of Military Time:

00:05 = 12:05 AM   12:00 = Noon
08:00 = 8:00 AM   20:45 = 8:45 PM

Emergency Contacts

Name _____ Phone _____ Mobile Phone _____

Name _____ Phone _____ Mobile Phone _____

Important Information:

Name _____ Phone _____

Carry this completed card with you for details of your employment location and emergency contacts.

PAIN ASSESSMENT TOOL

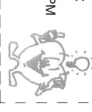

Ask the person to choose the face that best describes how much pain is present.

Blue Face '0'	Black Face '5'	Red Face '10'
NO PAIN	has some PAIN	Worst PAIN
(+1=Minimal)	(Moderate)	(Severe)

Ask questions to help identify the specific location and type of pain
(e.g., sharp, dull, throbbing, stabbing, aching, burning, nagging, unbearable)

©First Class Books, Inc.